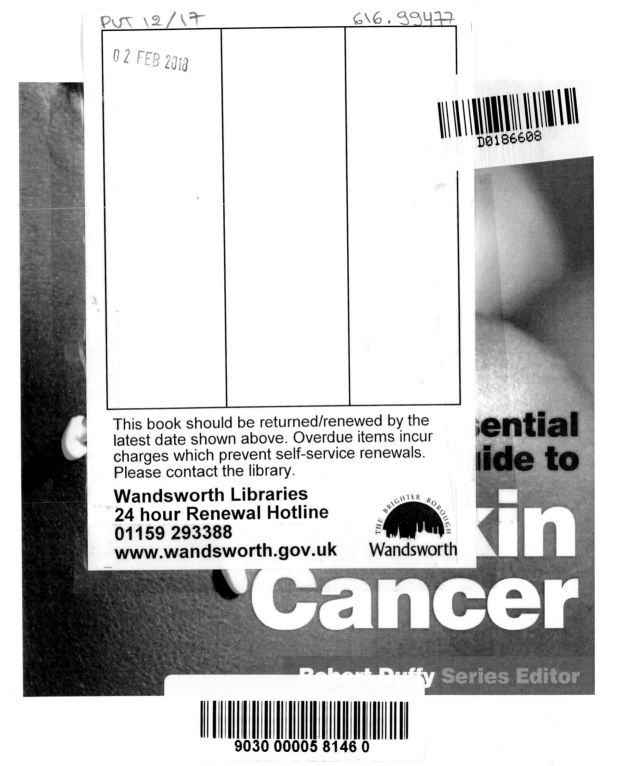

PUT 12/17

616.99477

sential
ide to
kin
Cancer

Robert Duffy Series Editor

Published in Great Britain in 2017 by

need2know

Remus House
Coltsfoot Drive
Peterborough
PE2 9BF
Telephone 01733 898103
www.need2knowbooks.co.uk

Contents

Introduction

S kin cancer is one of the most common forms of cancer in the UK and malignant melanoma – the most serious type – has become the most common form of cancer in young people aged 15 to 34. Even though the dangers of sunbathing and sunbed use are significantly linked to skin cancer, many people still don't do enough to protect their skin.

Many instances of skin cancer could be prevented if people took more notice of sun safety issues. In the UK, it's still often the norm to head off outside and sunbathe as soon as the sun comes out, and people often don't realise that skin damage can occur even on cloudy summer days. Even though a wide variety of sunscreen products exist, there's often still confusion over how much to use, what SPF factor to choose and how often it should be applied.

This book aims to help put an end to the confusion and set the record straight. It explores the facts about skin cancer, the different types that exist – non-melanoma and malignant melanoma, how to recognise the symptoms and how it's treated. There's advice for people going through the trauma of skin cancer and for friends and family who are supporting them.

Rather than just looking at skin cancer and what happens if it occurs, the book also offers a practical and informative guide about how it can be prevented in the first place. Throughout the book you'll find plenty of tips and advice that you can take away and put into action, helping you build up your own sun safety strategy. There are chapters focusing on the major risk factors, on preventing skin cancer and one chapter devoted entirely to sunscreen.

As well as exploring how individuals can protect themselves from the risks of skin cancer, the book also delves into the issues of how schools and employers can protect children and workers. Many schools and employers are already offering support, guidance and practical measures to deal with sun safety issues, but more could be done to protect vulnerable people who find themselves out in the heat of the midday sun.

The true dangers of using a sunbed are covered too and as gaining a tan still seems to be desirable these days, the book also takes a look at the only truly safe way of getting a tan – fake tan.

No one is too young or too old to learn how to protect their skin, so this book is aimed at all ages.

Whether you've already been affected by skin cancer, or know someone who has, have just received a diagnosis of skin cancer, or are keen to do all you can to protect your skin or change your old sun habits, this book will equip you with the facts, guide you through the practicalities and improve your knowledge of both skin cancer and sun safety issues.

Disclaimer

This book is aimed at providing general information about skin cancer and sun safety and is not intended to replace professional medical advice. It can be used alongside medical advice, but anyone concerned about sun safety, moles or skin issues are strongly advised to consult a medical practitioner.

While every care has been taken to validate the contents of this guide, the author advises that she does not claim medical qualifications. Readers should always seek advice from a qualified medical practitioner about any skin concern.

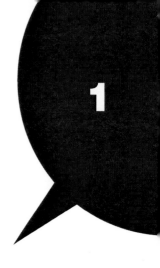

1

Understanding the Skin

To fully get to grips with the need for sun protection and some of the ways in which skin cancer occurs, we first need to understand the skin.

The structure and function of skin

It may come as a surprise to learn that the skin is the largest organ in the body and accounts for about 16% of our total body weight. Skin consists of three main layers:

- The epidermis – an elastic layer on the outside.
- The dermis – an inner layer.
- The subcutaneous layer – located under the dermis and made up of connective tissue and fat.

The epidermis is constantly being regenerated and it's the part of the skin where you find melanocytes, which produce the pigment known as melanin. Melanin is what gives the skin its colour and helps protect the skin from UV radiation.

The dermis, or inner layer, is where the sweat glands are located – these play a key role in regulating body temperature. The hair follicles are also found here, as well as the sebaceous glands which produce sebum oil to keep hairs free from bacteria.

The subcutaneous layer is found underneath the dermis and is the deepest layer of skin. It varies in size and thickness from individual to individual and consists of connective tissue (blood vessels and nerves), collagen and fat. It can act as an insulator, helping to conserve body heat and protect other internal organs from damage.

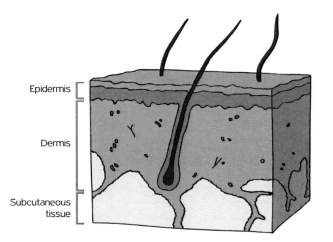

Epidermis

Dermis

Subcutaneous
tissue

What does skin do?

Skin has several major functions in keeping us healthy and free from harm.

The main functions are:

- To act as a protective barrier against injury.

- To prevent loss of moisture from the body.

- To help regulate body temperature.

- To act as an immune defence against infections.

- To produce vitamin D.

- To reduce the harmful effects of UV radiation.

- To act as a sensory organ, enabling us to touch things and feel hot or cold temperatures.

How does skin damage occur?

Damage to the skin starts from childhood and happens when the skin is exposed to the rays of the sun. The sun emits ultraviolet (UV) light, which consists of three different types of rays – UVA, UVB and UVC.

'People do need to spend some time in the sun as it's the most important source of vitamin D, which is important for good health. But it's important to remember that too much sun can lead to sunburn and skin cancer.'

Sara Hiom, director of health information, Cancer Research UK.

- UVA radiation is a long wavelength ray that can penetrate deep into the dermis (the inner layer). It affects the elastin in the skin and also ages the skin.

- UVB radiation is a shorter wavelength ray than UVA. It penetrates the epidermis (the upper layer) and can cause sunburn and skin cancer.

- UVC radiation cannot get through the ozone layer, so doesn't cause skin damage.

It used to be thought that only UVB exposure was linked to the development of skin cancer, but new evidence is highlighting the risks of UVA too. It's now believed that both UVA and UVB play a role in skin cancer as they both damage DNA.

To help people know when the sun's rays are particularly strong, the World Health Organisation developed the UV index. The index is used on weather reports and weather maps – it appears as a triangle with a number inside. The higher the number, the greater the UV level is.

It's often assumed that the effects of UV rays will only be felt on sunny days, but actually some UV can still get through on cloudy days too.

The impact of sun on skin

The sun has an impact on our skin in many different ways, with the most serious being skin cancer.

Exposure to some sunlight is important, as the skin uses it to produce vitamin D. Vitamin D is often called the 'sunshine vitamin' and it's involved in helping to build and maintain strong bones. Even though the sun has a positive effect by creating vitamin D, only a small amount of sun exposure is needed to build up our reserves of the vitamin.

When skin is exposed to sunlight, melanin – the pigment that gives skin its colour – is made and the skin becomes darker. This process is called getting a suntan, but rather than being a good thing, as most people assume, it's actually a sign that the skin has been damaged and is trying to protect itself. Sometimes the melanin is distributed unevenly on the skin and instead forms a freckle.

When UVA rays penetrate the skin deeply, this affects the elastin. The result is premature ageing, such as the development of wrinkles, brown pigmentation and saggy and leathery skin. The skin on younger people is damaged very easily in this way – and once the damage is done, it can't be reversed.

'Enjoying the sun safely while taking care not to burn should help people strike a balance between making enough vitamin D and avoiding a higher risk of skin cancer.'

Sara Hiom, director of health information, Cancer Research UK.

Getting to know your skin

In order to help protect against skin cancer, it's useful to get to know your skin. That means looking out for any freckles, moles or skin blemishes you have and knowing how your skin reacts in the sun, so you can apply sunscreen or cover up when necessary.

For example, you're more likely to burn easily if you have fair skin, fair hair, red hair or blue eyes. In contrast, if your skin is naturally darker, then you'll have more protection against burning. Getting burnt is not advisable, as sunburn is a major risk factor for skin cancer – in fact, it can double the risk.

Increased risk of skin cancer

Some people do have a higher risk of developing skin cancer, so if you fall into this category, it's even more important to take care of your skin and protect yourself when you're outside. Those with a higher risk generally have one or more of these characteristics:

- Lots of moles or freckles.
- Fair skin that burns very easily.
- Red or fair hair.
- A past experience of sunburn, especially when young.
- A past experience or a family history of skin cancer.

Brown or black skin

If you have naturally brown or black skin, then you'll have more melanin pigment in your skin cells. This helps protect the skin from the effects of UV rays and you'll have a lower chance of developing skin cancer.

However, this doesn't mean skin cancer definitely won't occur and people with brown or black skin do get skin cancer. In this instance, it's more likely to occur in areas of your skin that aren't exposed to the sun so often, such as the soles of your feet.

'People should try and get to know their own skin. This means understanding your skin type and knowing how likely you are to burn. Everyone is different, but you're more at risk from melanoma if you have fair skin, red hair, lots of freckles, moles or a family history of the disease.'

Sara Hiom, director of health information, Cancer Research UK.

Looking out for skin changes

Once you've got to know your skin, you can keep an eye out for any changes that occur, both with new or existing moles and other areas of your skin.

Moles

Moles are small dark marks that appear on the skin, almost anywhere on the body. They're usually brown in colour, but it's also normal to have darker moles or ones that are almost the same colour as your skin. Moles are usually circular or oval in their shape and about the size and diameter of an average pencil. As far as the look of a mole is concerned, they can be smooth, rough, raised, flat or even hairy!

Many people are born with moles and have them throughout their life, but moles can also appear at any time. Moles tend to develop during the first 20 years of life, but they can appear during a person's 30s and 40s. They're particularly likely to occur if you spend a lot of time in the sun and may appear on the areas of your body that are most exposed to sunlight.

It's not unusual for moles to change slightly over time, for example in colour, shape or size, and many mole changes are completely harmless. For example, changes in the colour of a mole are often due to a benign increase in the pigment cells in the skin.

However, a small number can develop into skin cancer, so to be on the safe side it's good to know where on your body your moles are located and to check them regularly.

Skin

Changes to your skin can occur due to hormones, particularly during pregnancy, and in many cases may be totally harmless. However, if you suddenly find that you have a patch of skin or a freckle that's itchy, tender, bleeding, flaky, oozing or red, and there's no obvious cause for it (such as an allergic reaction or skin condition, like eczema), then see your GP.

Try to check your skin once a month and look from head to feet, even between the toes and the soles of your feet. For awkward or hard-to-see areas, like your back, try looking in mirrors where this is feasible or ask someone else to check for you, especially where you have any known moles.

'Many of the signs and symptoms that could suggest cancer often turn out to reveal a much less serious ailment. But it's better to play safe, so if you notice a change in the size, shape or colour of a mole or other patch of skin, it's a good idea to get it checked out by a GP.'

Sara Hiom, director of health information, Cancer Research UK.

Checking moles – what to look for

When you're checking your moles, some of the signs to look out for include:

- A new mole that looks different or unusual.
- An existing mole that has suddenly grown in size, over weeks or months.
- A mole that has a ragged or uneven edge.
- A mole that feels painful, uncomfortable or itchy.
- A mole that has varying shades of different colours in it.
- A mole that has an inflamed or red edge.
- A mole that is bleeding, oozing or has become crusty.

You can also use the so-called ABCD rule to assess your moles, the standard used by doctors:

- Asymmetry – the two halves of your mole don't look the same.
- Border – the edges of your mole are blurred, jagged or irregular.
- Colour – the colour of your mole is not the same throughout, with more than one shade.
- Diameter – your mole is wider than 6mm in diameter, or wider than the size of an average pencil.

'My aunt and grandmother have both had skin cancer and I know how horrible it is. Now I regularly check my moles for changes, as catching it quickly can make a difference.'

Helen

Asymmetry

Border

Colour

Diameter

If any of your moles match these descriptions or fit into the ABCD rule, then it's advisable to see your GP – if only to get it checked out for your peace of mind.

When to see your GP

If you've taken to regularly checking your moles and the rest of your skin and notice any changes or new patches of skin that look different, then see your GP without delay. In many cases, the changes may turn out to be perfectly normal, but it's better to be safe and sure that it's all fine, than leave it unchecked.

If you don't get things checked out and it turns out to be skin cancer, leaving it for longer could mean that the cancer is more advanced or harder to treat.

Checklist

- Have you ever been sunburnt?
- Do you know what type of skin you have and whether you burn easily?
- Do you keep an eye on the UV index on the weather forecast?
- Do you know where on your body you have moles?
- How often do you check your skin and moles?

Summing Up

- Skin is made up of three layers – the epidermis, the dermis and the subcutaneous layer – and it's the largest organ in the body. Skin has several key functions, including helping protect us from injury and infection, regulating body temperature, producing vitamin D and preventing loss of moisture from the body.

- Skin damage can begin from childhood and is caused by the skin being exposed to the rays of the sun. The UV light emitted from the sun is made up of three types of rays – UVA, UVB and UVC. Both UVA and UVB play a role in skin damage and skin cancer.

- In addition to skin cancer, exposure to the sun produces vitamin D which is good for us. It also causes us to suntan when melanin darkens, affects the elastin and causes premature ageing. Although many people associate suntans with a healthy look, they're in fact a sign that the skin has been damaged. Experiencing sunburn can double the risk of skin cancer.

- In order to help protect your skin and spot any changes early on, it's helpful to get to know your skin and what's normal for you. Look out for skin changes and mole changes on a monthly basis and see your GP if you're concerned.

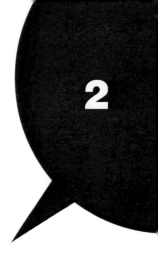

2

Risk Factors for Skin Cancer

To understand some of the reasons why skin cancer occurs, it's important to look at the risk factors involved – some of which we have a degree of control over.

Who is at most risk of skin cancer?

'The British weather does cause a problem. For a lot of the time we see no sun and so when it does come out, people want to make the most of it and may not take as much care to avoid burning as they should.'

Sara Hiom, director of health information, Cancer Research UK.

Anyone can potentially develop skin cancer, especially if they abuse their skin by spending a lot of time sunbathing, using sunbeds and not worrying about wearing sunscreen, but there are some people who have a higher risk to start with. For these people, it's even more important that they take care of their skin, recognise the risks and do their best to reduce their risk.

As covered in chapter 1, those with a higher risk of skin cancer will be able to say 'yes' to one or more of these factors:

- Having lots of moles or freckles.
- Having fair skin that is prone to burning very easily.
- Having red or fair hair.
- Having had a past experience of sunburn, especially when young (even one bad episode of sunburn increases the skin cancer risk).
- Having had a past experience of skin cancer, or knowledge that skin cancer runs in the family.

How sun damage starts

Sun damage starts from a young age, as soon as the skin is exposed to sunlight. Put simply, the skin becomes damaged by the sun if you don't take steps to protect it.

It's not possible to see the UV rays from the sun, but as the sun shines it emits UVA and UVB rays which beat down onto anything in their way – including humans and our skin. There are also UVC rays, but these don't make it through the ozone layer and are not linked to skin cancer.

UVA has long wavelength rays and can penetrate deep into our skin causing skin damage, affecting the elastin in the skin and increasing premature ageing. UVB has shorter wavelength rays, penetrating the outer layers of the skin, and is a big factor in causing sunburn.

Both forms of UVA and UVB radiation can damage the cells of the skin and cause skin cancer. Inside the nucleus of the cells, the DNA, or genetic code, is carried, and this can be harmed by the effects of the sun.

Although it's traditionally been thought fashionable to have a tan, in reality a suntan signifies that your skin has suffered damage.

The effects of binge sunbathing

Spending day after day lying in the hot sun or indulging in bouts of binge sunbathing isn't a good move for your skin, yet people still do it. But it's not just the hardcore binge sunbathers who should be worried.

Even if you don't normally sunbathe but like to make the most of the sun while you're on holiday, this can be detrimental to your skin. If you have short and intensive periods of time when your skin is exposed to the sun, especially if you end up experiencing burning, then this can increase the risk of malignant melanoma – the most serious form of skin cancer.

If you get sunburnt, the skin reacts by causing redness, pain and inflammation. Your skin becomes hot and it can be painful, in severe cases you can also end up with blisters and swelling.

After the bad effects of sunburn have passed, the skin reacts by getting rid of its damaged cells – or what we know as peeling. Even though the damaged layer of skin peels and flakes away, leaving room for new skin layers to be produced, some of the effects of the sunburn damage will still remain and can cause problems in the future.

Basically, sunburn is not good for your skin in the short or long term, and should be avoided.

Are babies and children at risk?

Babies and children have thin, delicate skin that is easily damaged and because of this they are at risk from the effects of the sun.

Although skin cancer is rare in babies and children, it's the long-term effects that can be a problem. Skin cancer can take years to develop, but the damage to the DNA in the skin cells when babies are young is stored up and can subsequently develop into skin cancer later in life.

Research has shown that being sunburnt during childhood is linked to an increased risk of skin cancer later in life. Some experts even suggest that the risk of malignant melanoma is doubled by having just one instance of sunburn that blisters before you reach the age of 20.

Although skin cancer may seem like something that only affects people in later life, and gives youngsters the idea that they're immune to it, teenagers are in fact at risk too.

'Although a tan may seem desirable, it's really just a sign that your skin has been damaged.'

For example, teenagers often yearn to get a tan and make the most of laying out in the sun when it's hot, yet malignant melanoma – the most serious form of skin cancer – is the most common cancer in those aged between 15 and 34 years old. Although a tan may seem desirable, it's really just a sign that your skin has been damaged, and with the risk of skin cancer increasing when you suffer from sunburn, is it really worth it?

Genetic risk factors

Genetics and family histories of diseases can often play a part in your own risk of developing cancer. Those who have a family history of melanoma are believed to have about double the risk of developing skin cancer themselves, compared to those without the family link.

If one of your parents has had squamous cell skin cancer (see chapter 3 for more information), then Cancer Research UK suggests you may have a two to three times higher than average risk of getting it too.

In some cases, there are particular genes that can be passed through generations of families, increasing the genetic predisposition and risk of getting skin cancer.

Plus, your skin type – which is of course passed on from your parents – can be a risk factor in skin cancer as well, with those with pale, light or freckled skin being particularly at risk of burning from the sun.

Other risk factors

There are a few other potential risk factors for skin cancer, although many of these are rare.

Weak immune systems

People who are on medication that may weaken their immune system, called immunosuppressant drugs, may have a slightly increased risk of getting skin cancer. However, medical experts say that the need to take the immunosuppressants, such as after having had a kidney transplant, outweighs the risk of skin cancer.

Exposure to chemicals

In rare cases, extreme exposure to certain chemicals, for example in a working environment, could cause non-melanoma cancer. Some of the potential chemicals that could do this include:

- Coal tar.
- Soot.
- Asphalt.
- Creosote.
- Arsenic.
- Parrafin wax.
- Petroleum derivatives.
- Hair dye.

Radiotherapy

People who've previously had radiotherapy treatment, for example to treat skin cancer or another form of cancer, may potentially be at risk from skin cancer later in life. The skin cancer may form in the area where they had the radiotherapy.

All about UV and its effects

As covered in chapter 1, UVA has long wavelength radiation which means that it can get deep into the skin, affecting elastin and causing an ageing effect. Although it was previously thought that UVA might not play a part in the development of skin cancer, more recent research has suggested it does.

UVB has shorter wavelength radiation and only gets into the upper layer of the skin, but it can have major effects. It's responsible for sunburn and can cause skin cancer.

UVC does not penetrate the ozone layer, so it is not a skin concern factor.

The strength of UV rays depends on a variety of factors including:

- The time of day.

- The time of year.

- Where in the world you're located.

- The weather.

- How high up you are (at higher altitudes the UV can be stronger than lower points).

The UV index was developed by the World Health Organisation to represent the risk present in the sun rays. The greater the number, the higher the risk and the less time it takes for the sun to cause skin damage.

The UV index is incorporated into weather reports, particularly during the hot summer months, so you may well see a weather map with the UV index included. The symbol to look out for is a triangle with a number inside. You can also find the UV index weather reports all year round on the Met Office website – see www.metoffice.gov.uk.

Types of skin cancer

There are two main types of skin cancer – non-melanoma skin cancer and malignant melanoma skin cancer.

Non-melanoma is the most common type of skin cancer and experts believe it could account for at least 100,000 cases in the UK each year. There are two main types of non-melanoma skin cancer:

- Basal cell carcinoma.

- Squamous cell carcinoma.

Both of these non-melanoma skin cancers are explored in more depth in chapter 3.

Malignant melanoma is the most serious form of skin cancer, although it's also the least common. It's rare in children, but it's worryingly become the most common cancer for those aged 15 to 34 to be diagnosed with – which may well be linked to the prevalence and love of sunbathing and tanning.

You can read more about malignant melanoma in chapter 4.

Myths about skin cancer and sun damage

Myths about skin cancer and sun damage continue to exist, which doesn't help with people's understanding of what is correct and incorrect. Here are some of the common skin cancer and sun safety myths and the true facts behind them.

Myth

Sunscreen is all the protection you need against the effects of the sun.

Fact

Although sunscreen is an important part of the fight against the harmful effects of the sun, and something that everyone should include in their sun safety routine, it is not the only precaution you should take.

In addition to using sunscreen, you should learn to stay out of the heat of the strong midday sun, sit in the shade, wear a hat and cover up exposed areas of your body with suitable clothing.

Myth

It's safer to tan using a sunbed than lying out in the sun and sunbathing.

Fact

This is a dreadful myth, as a sunbed is certainly not a safe option. In fact, there's no safe method of getting a tan – other than using fake tan – as both sunbeds and sunbathing increase the risk of skin cancer.

'Research has shown that being sunburnt during childhood is linked to an increased risk of skin cancer later in life.'

Myth

I'm not at risk from sun damage as I don't sunbathe.

Fact

While it's true that getting sunburnt can increase your risk of skin cancer and is something that sunbathing devotees may suffer from, not sunbathing doesn't automatically make you immune to all sun damage. Sun damage builds up over time, and the sun can damage your skin at any time when you're outdoors without wearing sunscreen or protecting your skin.

Myth

It's too late to start protecting my skin now, as damage must have already occurred.

Fact

If you have been a lifelong fan of sunbathing or have frequently used tanning beds, then the chances are that damage will have been done to your skin. However, this is no excuse for not protecting your skin now as it can make a difference.

Checklist

- Be aware about how sun damage starts.
- Don't be tempted by binge sunbathing.
- Take care of babies' and children's skin.
- If you have a potentially higher risk factor of skin cancer, don't ignore the risks and take extra care to protect your skin.
- Make sure you're clued up about what's true and what's not when it comes to skin cancer and sun damage.

Summing Up

- Anyone could be at risk of skin cancer, especially if you don't take steps to protect your skin from the harmful effects of the sun.

- Sun damage can occur from an early age and occurs when unprotected skin is exposed to the UV rays of the sun.

- On the surface of it, sunbathing may seem like a fun activity to take part in, but in fact it can prove dangerous for your skin. Binge sunbathing or staying out in the sun for hours at a time isn't recommended and could do significant harm, especially if you get sunburnt.

- No one is immune to the effects of the sun. Babies and children have very delicate skin which can easily be damaged by the sun – and this skin damage is stored and builds up over the years.

- The sun isn't the only risk factor involved in skin cancer. Sometimes genetic factors play a part, or people may succumb due to a weak immune system or exposure to particular chemicals.

- The UV light emitted contains UVA and UVB rays, which both play a part in the development of skin cancer.

- The two main types of skin cancer are non-melanoma and malignant melanoma – the latter is the more serious type.

- There are still a lot of myths about skin cancer and sun damage floating around. It's wise to check if they are really true before believing everything you may hear.

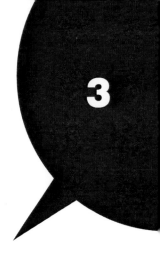

3

Non-melanoma Skin Cancer

on-melanoma is the most common type of skin cancer. Statistics from Cancer Research UK indicate that in 2006 over 81,600 incidents of non-melanoma skin cancer were registered. Experts believe this isn't the complete picture though, as not all cases are reported, and the reality is more likely to be at least 100,000 cases in the UK each year.

Basal cell carcinoma

Basal cell carcinoma is the most common form of non-melanoma skin cancer in the UK, accounting for over 75% of all skin cancer cases. It's called basal cell carcinoma as the cancer starts in the deep basal cell layer of the epidermis – the outer layer of the skin.

In most cases, basal cell carcinomas grow slowly and rarely spread to other parts of the body. However, it's important that they're treated as if left untreated, they can cause even more skin damage and form into an ulcer – what is known as a rodent ulcer.

Basal cell carcinomas are most commonly found on the face, ears, hands, shoulders, back and scalp.

Squamous cell carcinoma

Squamous cell carcinoma is the second most common form of skin cancer in the UK.

This form of non-melanoma cancer occurs in the outermost cells of the skin, when cells grow out of control and form a tumour. It can occur on any part of your body, but it's most likely to happen in areas of the skin that have had a lot of exposure to the sun, such as the neck, head, face, lips, ears, arms, shoulders, legs and hands.

In addition, this type of cancer can occur on areas of the skin that have previously been damaged through burning, scarring, ulcers, wounds or even from x-rays.

If left untreated, squamous cell carcinomas can spread to other parts of your body.

Causes of non-melanoma skin cancer

The most common causes of non-melanoma skin cancer is too much exposure to UV light – either from the sun or from sunbeds.

Other factors that can increase the risk of non-melanoma cancer include:

- Having lots of moles or freckles.

- Having fair skin that burns easily.

- Having red or fair hair.

- A past experience of sunburn, especially when young.

- Having previously had a non-melanoma skin cancer, or if a history of it runs in your family.

With squamous cell carcinoma, you could also be at an increased risk if you've had UV light treatment for certain skin conditions, such as psoriasis, or if your immune system has been affected by medication after an organ transplant or treatment for leukaemia.

The symptoms of non-melanoma cancer

Basal cell carcinoma is usually painless and the first sign can be the appearance of a small, slow-growing, shiny pink or red lump. Other signs include a scab that bleeds on and off and doesn't heal, changes to your skin (like a scar changing or patch of scaly skin similar to eczema) or a small sore that has white raised edges. If left, it's the latter type of sore with raised edges that could get worse and form an ulcer, or rodent ulcer.

With squamous cell carcinoma, which grows at a faster rate than basal cell carcinoma, it may at first look like a scaly patch of eczema, a crusty area of skin, a pink lump or a red and inflamed sore. It's common for them to have scaly or hard skin on the surface and they can easily start bleeding or begin to form into an ulcer.

For both, the main signs to look out for are:

- Sore lumps, bumps or patches that appear, but don't get any better.

- Sore lumps, bumps or patches that grow bigger.

The treatment of non-melanoma skin cancer is generally easier the earlier it's detected, so if you do spot any changes to your skin, it's important to get them checked by your GP as soon as possible.

How is non-melanoma skin cancer diagnosed?

If you're worried about an area of your skin and have noticed changes that you're concerned about, then the first port of call should be a visit to your GP.

If your GP suspects that a basal cell carcinoma or squamous cell carcinoma could be the cause, or if your GP wants to rule them out as causes, then the likely scenario is that you'll be referred to a dermatologist.

The only way of knowing for certain if it is a non-melanoma skin cancer is for a sample of the skin to be taken and examined under a microscope. The procedure – a biopsy – is usually undertaken with the help of a local anaesthetic, which deadens the area in question, but it does partly depend on where the problem is and its size.

There are four main types of biopsy:

- A shave biopsy – where the top layer of the skin in the affected area is taken off for analysis.

- A punch biopsy – where a thicker layer of skin, including deeper tissues, is removed.

- An incisional biopsy – where a small piece of the lump or tumour is removed with a surgical knife. This will require stitches, which may well be soluble (i.e. dissolve after a week to 10 days).

- An excisional biopsy – where the whole of the lump or tumour is removed. This will also require stitches and they may be soluble.

Once your skin sample has been taken during the biopsy, it will be taken off to a laboratory to be analysed closely under a microscope.

You won't receive the results immediately – it will probably be about a two to three week wait – and you'll either go back to see a dermatologist for the results or be given them by your GP.

Treatment options

There are various types of treatment available for non-melanoma cancer and it depends, in part, on the type of cancer you have, the size of the basal cell or squamous cell carcinoma, where on your body it's located and how long you've had it.

Surgery

The most common form of treatment is surgery to remove the carcinoma.

In cases where the cancer is small, you may only require a local anaesthetic while surgery is performed to cut away the carcinoma and some of the non-affected skin immediately surrounding it. It's important to remove some of the skin around a tumour so this can be analysed. Hopefully it will prove to be healthy, but if it contains any cancer cells then more treatment might be required.

In the case of larger cancers, a general anaesthetic may be required. You may also need a skin graft too, to help patch up the area where the cancer has been removed.

The skin graft can be done under local or general anaesthetic and involves removing a small piece of skin from a donor site on your body. This is usually chosen from somewhere that doesn't get seen too often or won't be obvious to other people, such as your inner thigh. When the skin is taken, it will leave a mark a bit like a graze and it will be a bit uncomfortable while it heals, but the skin will grow back quite quickly, often within a matter of weeks.

Sometimes a more complicated repair, called a skin flap, is performed. The flap is a thicker piece of skin tissue than a skin graft and is removed complete with the skin and the tissue below it, so it has its own blood supply.

Skin flaps are taken from areas close to the tumour wound and are usually used for situations where the scar would be very noticeable, such as on the face. It's a complicated form of surgery, but it can have a better end result than a skin graft.

Photodynamic therapy

Photodynamic therapy, or PDT, is a newer form of treatment that offers an alternative to having surgery and can be carried out in the outpatient department at hospitals.

With PDT, you either have a special light sensitising cream put on the area of skin where the cancer is, or you're given an injection or drug to take (the active ingredient is called 5-aminolaevulinic acid, or 5-ALA). The cream, injection or drug will make your skin sensitive to light.

It takes from three to six hours for the cream, injection or drug to be properly absorbed by the skin and the area of your skin has to be covered while it's working. When it's properly absorbed, a laser light is shone onto the affected area of skin for up to 45 minutes at a time. The laser light will kill off any cells that have been absorbed by the drug.

The therapy is only appropriate for certain forms of cancer, where the skin cancer isn't too deep or there are several carcinomas in one area. It's not suitable for squamous cell skin cancer, or deeper skin cancers, as the light can't get through the skin to a deep enough level to do any good.

Curettage and cautery

With curettage and cautery, the carcinoma is first scraped away (a process known as curettage) and then the skin surface is sealed up (known as cautery). Sometimes the process is known as 'C and C'.

This can be used for small basal cell carcinomas and squamous cell carcinomas, but it is only suitable if the cancer is small. It's performed as day surgery, with local anaesthetic, and the affected skin is scraped away or scooped off with a spoon shaped instrument called a curette. In order to stop the wound from bleeding, it's cauterised with an electrosurgical unit.

After you've had this procedure, the area will need to be kept dry for several days, to allow it to heal. Ideally, the wound area should be kept uncovered and exposed to air, but you will be advised if you need to wear any dressings. When the local anaesthetic has worn off, it can initially be painful, but pain-killers can help relieve the discomfort.

A scab will form and after 10 to 14 days it should peel away naturally. With any procedure like this, where the skin is cut away, it's hard to avoid scarring, so you may be left with some marks on your skin. In most cases, they are similar to the size of the original skin cancer.

Cryotherapy

Cryotherapy (also called cryosurgery) is a treatment that uses cold liquid nitrogen to destroy the cancer cells and tissue by freezing.

It's often used if a carcinoma is very small or only affects the surface layers of the skin. Liquid nitrogen is sprayed onto the affected area to freeze the cancer. It's cold and can feel a bit uncomfortable – a bit like being stung by a bee – and afterwards the skin may continue to feel a bit delicate.

A few days after you've had the treatment, a blister may appear containing fluid or blood. Any fluid needs to be drained off by a doctor, but the aim is to leave the top of the blister intact.

The area is covered with a dressing until a scab forms. In time, the scab will drop off and the cancer cells should have been removed. You may end up with a small scar in the affected area.

Surgery to remove lymph nodes

Squamous cell cancer can sometimes spread to other parts of your body, so if doctors think there's the possibility that it has spread to your nearby lymph nodes, then you may need to have surgery to remove them.

This is important; if cancer cells spread to your lymph nodes, they could grow into secondary tumours and spread from the lymph nodes into other parts of your body.

The lymphatic system in the body is one of the ways in which the body helps fight infection. It's made up of organs, such as the spleen and bone marrow, and lymph nodes, or lymph glands, and they're connected by lots of tiny lymphatic vessels. The lymph nodes are small, kidney bean shaped organs, situated in various parts of the body, including in the armpits, neck and groin. Fluid that travels through the lymph nodes is filtered to remove bacteria or dying cells, but sometimes they can become affected with cancer cells.

The most common sign that the lymph nodes have become affected by cancer is if the lymph nodes suddenly become larger or feel hard to touch (although they can also react in this way from infections). Sometimes an indication comes up on an ultrasound, MRI or CT scan, or if the affected lymph nodes are in the chest or abdomen, they may cause symptoms such as breathlessness or backache.

If there are only a small number of cancer cells in the lymph nodes, it's harder for doctors to be sure and the only way is to remove part or all of the lymph nodes.

Lymph node surgery, or lymphadenectomy, is a major form of surgery and you will need to stay in hospital for a few days. The surgery is normally performed under general anaesthetic and, depending on where the cells are being removed from, lasts for about 45 minutes. A small cut is made over the lymph nodes, the nodes are removed and the area is stitched up again.

Afterwards you will feel sore and painful for a while, especially after the effects of the anaesthetic have worn off, and may need to take pain-killers to control the pain. Your doctor or consultant will advise you more about how long your recovery will take, but in general you're advised not to drive until you feel confident that you'll be able to perform an emergency stop if you need to and to avoid strenuous exercise or lifting for a few weeks.

Radiotherapy

Radiotherapy is sometimes used to treat skin cancer, particularly if surgery isn't suitable. It's also used after surgery to reduce the likelihood of the cancer returning.

This treatment involves using high energy rays to destroy the carcinoma and is given at the radiotherapy unit in hospital. It's only aimed at the area of skin with the cancer cells and is good for non-melanoma in awkward areas, areas where other treatment may cause long-term damage, like the face, or for tumours that are deep in the skin.

Sometimes only a single treatment is all that is needed to clear the cancer, but in other cases a course of treatment over several weeks, given once a day from Monday to Friday, may be required.

Initially, it can seem like the treatment is doing more harm than good, as the skin can become very red, sore and inflamed. But rest assured that the skin will consequently dry up and form into a crust or scab. Eventually the scab will fall away and there'll be new, healed skin underneath.

Compared to chemotherapy, there are fewer side effects, although your skin in the area being treated can become sore. Depending on the part of your body being treated, some side effects can occur immediately after the treatment, but you will be advised by your doctor before the treatment starts. Although radiotherapy generally doesn't cause hair loss, it can sometimes occur in the area of the body being treated, but it is usually only temporary.

It's normal to feel tired and emotional after having radiotherapy treatment and ideally you should give yourself time to rest after treatments. The exact recovery time will vary from person to person and depends on how long the course of treatment lasts.

Chemotherapy

Chemotherapy is occasionally used to treat early stage basal or squamous cell non-melanoma cancers.

Topical chemotherapy uses a cream, which usually contains a drug known as 5-fluorouracil or 5FU, applied directly to the skin. This is something that can be carried out at home and you will be given details of how to do it from a doctor or specialist nurse.

Treatment with chemotherapy cream can make the skin very red and sore, and any exposure to sun can make this worse, but after the treatment is finished it should calm down in a few weeks.

In rare cases where squamous cell cancer has spread to other parts of the body, then it may be necessary to be given full chemotherapy treatment with intravenous injections.

Checklist

- If you're worried about a mole or a patch of unusual skin, don't delay – see your GP as soon as possible.

- If you're diagnosed with non-melanoma skin cancer, don't be afraid to ask questions if you don't understand what's going to happen.

- Ask about the treatment you'll receive, how long treatment is likely to last and what you can expect.

Summing Up

- Non-melanoma is the most common type of skin cancer. There are two main types – basal cell carcinoma, which accounts for over 75% of all cases, and squamous cell carcinoma.

- Basal cell carcinoma occurs in the basal cell layer of the epidermis and squamous cell cancer starts in the outermost cells of the skin.

- Non-melanoma cancer is most commonly caused by too much exposure to UV light, through sunbathing or using sunbeds. But it's also possible to have an increased risk if you have fair skin that burns easily, have lots of moles or freckles, have a history of it in your family or if you've suffered bad sunburn when you were younger.

- The main signs to look out for are changes to your skin, such as sore lumps, bumps or patches that appear and don't get better, or get bigger. The main way of determining if it is non-melanoma cancer is to have a biopsy, where a small area of skin is taken away for testing.

- There are various types of treatment options available for non-melanoma skin cancer. Cases are judged on an individual basis, so you get the most appropriate treatment for yourself. The choice of treatment depends on the type of cancer, the size of the tumour, where it's located on the body and how long it's likely to have been there.

- Many small forms of non-melanoma, caught in the early stages, can be successfully removed with minimal effects. However, if squamous cell cancer has spread to your lymph nodes, it runs the risk of spreading to other parts of your body, and it may be necessary to have surgery to remove the lymph nodes.

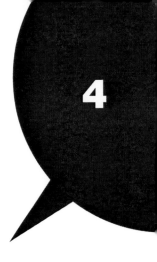

4

Malignant Melanoma Skin Cancer

M alignant melanoma is the most serious type of skin cancer and it's also the least common form of skin cancer. In 2006, over 10,400 new cases were diagnosed in the UK – 5,607 in women and 4,803 in men. It is the sixth most common cancer in females. Even though the risk of malignant melanoma increases with age, it is the most common cancer for those aged 15 to 34.

What is malignant melanoma?

Malignant melanoma is a type of skin cancer that can start in either a mole or an area of skin that looks normal.

It develops from cells called melanocytes, which are found between the dermis and epidermis layers of the skin. Their usual job is to make the pigment or colour of our skin, which helps protect the body from the UV light of the sun.

However, when malignant melanoma occurs, the melanocytes grow and divide much faster than normal and spread to the upper layers of the skin. The effect of this rapid cell growth can cause a mole or a dark spot to appear on your skin.

According to Cancer Research UK, the estimated lifetime risk of developing malignant melanoma is 1 in 91 for men and 1 in 77 for women in the UK.

Types of malignant melanoma

There are four main types of malignant melanoma.

Superficial spreading melanoma

This is the most common type of malignant melanoma in the UK, accounting for 70% of cases and it most frequently affects people aged 30-50. It's normally larger than 6mm in size, has irregular or asymmetrical borders, can be flat or slightly elevated and have various colours in it, including brown, black, blue, pink or even white.

This melanoma starts slowly by growing out over the surface of the skin, rather than downwards. If it's caught early, it's not at risk of spreading – if it isn't caught, it can then grow down into the skin. It usually starts on the legs for women and on the back or chest for men.

Nodula melanoma

This type of malignant melanoma is the second most common and is a cancer that usually affects middle-aged people. It can grow on a faster basis than other forms and is most often found on the head, neck, back and chest, as well as areas of the skin that haven't been exposed to much sun. If it's not removed, it can quickly begin to grow downwards into the skin.

It can start off by looking very dark brown or black in colour and can develop from both moles and areas of the skin that were otherwise fine.

Lentigo maligna melanoma

This is a malignant melanoma that normally affects older people, particularly anyone who's been a sun worshipper or had a lot of exposure to the sun over the years due to spending a lot of time outside. It can develop from pigmented areas of the skin, known as lentigo maligna, and can slowly get bigger or change shape over the years.

It may look irregular in shape, be flat, dark brown, black or variegated in colour; it may form lumps, or nodules, as it grows deeper into the skin. It commonly starts on the neck or face and grows very slowly. It accounts for about 10% of all melanomas.

Acral lentiginous melanoma

Acral melanoma is very rare and most often affects people with black or brown skin. Unlike other melanomas, it's not thought to be linked to sun exposure. It usually occurs in areas such as the soles of the feet, palms of the hands, toe nails or even under the nails, and can start off looking like a brown or black discolouration or a streak of discoloured skin.

Although malignant melanoma is most commonly associated with the skin, there are other rare forms that grow in other areas of the body, including in the internal organs and in the eye.

The symptoms of malignant melanoma

Like non-malignant melanoma, one of the common symptoms that can indicate a problem is a sudden change in an existing mole or freckle on your skin.

'Most melanoma skin cancers are caused by over exposure to UV rays. But, crucially, if people are careful not to redden or burn, especially if they have fair, freckly or moley skin, then most cases of malignant melanoma could be prevented.'

Sara Hiom, director of health information, Cancer Research UK.

As mentioned earlier, the ABCD mole rule can be used to help identify any changes.

- Asymmetry – melanomas are often asymmetrical or irregular in shape.

- Border – melanomas are likely to have an irregular border, with jagged edges rather than smooth.

- Colour – melanomas commonly have more than one colour. For example, they may have different shades of brown, as well as black, red, pink, white or even blue areas.

- Diameter – melanomas can be quite large and over 6mm in diameter.

It's also worth adding an extra E to your melanoma mole symptom list, which stands for evolving. If the mole is evolving and changing, whether it be in size, shape, colour, texture or how it feels (if it's tingling, itching, bleeding or crusting), then it's important to get it checked out by your GP.

However, half of all malignant melanomas also develop from an area of skin that used to be perfectly normal. When this happens, it can look like a dark brown or black area, or as if an unusual looking new mole has appeared. If anything like this suddenly appears on your skin, and you're not sure why or what it is, then it's important to have it examined.

The causes of malignant melanoma

Like non-melanoma skin cancer, a common cause of malignant melanoma is too much exposure to UV light from the sun, through sunbathing or using a sunbed. In fact, statistics show that people with malignant melanoma are twice as likely to have suffered bad sunburn at least once in their life, and the risk of melanoma is even higher if you've been sunburnt on multiple occasions.

There are other risk factors too and these include:

- Having fair skin that burns easily (and also red hair, fair hair, blue eyes or freckles).

- Having lots of moles – if you have over 100 moles, then you're deemed to be at a greater risk of getting skin cancer.

- Having moles that are large or an atypical (irregular) shape can also pose an increased risk.

- Having a family history of melanoma – if you have two or more close relatives who've had skin cancer, then your risk is higher. Research is continuing into whether a faulty gene could be inherited by families and be increasing the risk of skin cancer.

- Where you were born. People who have fair skin and were born in hot countries, such as Australia, have an increased risk of melanoma, as they may well have had more exposure to the sun when they were very young.

If for any reason you have a weak immune system, for example due to taking immunosuppressants after an organ transplant or if you have HIV, then this can also put you at a greater risk of developing melanoma.

Even though having black or brown skin lowers the risk of getting melanoma, it doesn't mean you'll never be at risk.

How is it diagnosed?

It's important to try to find, diagnose and treat malignant melanoma as soon as possible because if it isn't removed, the cancerous cells can go deeper into the layers of the skin. If it gets into the blood vessels or lymph nodes then it can spread to other parts of the body.

If you've found an area of your skin that you're worried about, noticed changes to moles or discovered new suspicious moles that have developed suddenly, then do go to see your GP.

If your GP thinks the mole or skin looks suspicious, then they will refer you to a specialist centre. A biopsy is the only accurate test available to correctly diagnose malignant melanoma and they may do this as the first course of action.

Although people with suspected non-malignant melanoma often have their moles removed under local anaesthetic at the GP's surgery, with suspected cases of malignant melanoma, the guidelines from the National Institute for Health and Clinical Excellence (NICE) state that you should be referred to a specialist centre within two weeks of seeing a GP.

Sometimes, after referral, a dermatoscopy test will be done to examine the area of skin in more detail first. It's pain-free and involves some oil being put onto your skin, before a dermatoscope is used by the doctor to look at your skin. It's a bit

'With the rates of malignant melanoma in the UK rising faster than any other cancer, it's more important than ever that people are aware of the dangers of getting burnt, either in the sun or from using sunbeds.'

Sara Hiom, director of health information, Cancer Research UK.

like a magnifying glass and magnifies the area by up to 10 times, so the doctor can see it in much more detail than the naked eye could manage. Depending on what they find, the next step after this may well be a biopsy.

The biopsy

The biopsy is usually carried out under local anaesthetic, although this can depend on where the mole is located – awkward places may result in the need for general anaesthetic. An injection is given into the skin to make the area numb, then the doctor will cut away the mole, or the area of skin being investigated, before putting in some stitches. The mole/skin sample is sent away to a laboratory for testing.

Sometimes the stitches need to be taken out if they're not soluble, and you may well have them taken out at the same time as collecting your biopsy results. If everything turns out to be normal, then no further action is needed. However, in the case of cancerous or pre-cancerous cells being detected, you will need more tests or treatment.

One of the most important issues is whether or not the biopsy removes all the cancerous cells from the skin affected, or if some are still left behind. If there are still cancerous or pre-cancerous cells lurking in your skin, these could go on to develop full blown melanoma or spread to other parts of your body.

Medical experts will look closely at the skin tissue that was removed to make sure that a healthy margin of skin tissue exists around it. If it does, all the cancer cells should have been removed, but if it doesn't, and cancer cells could be left behind, more surgery will be needed. In this case, you'll need to have an operation called a wide local excision.

Wide local excision

The wide local excision is designed to take away any other cancerous or pre-cancerous cells. It's usually conducted under local anaesthetic in hospital, although sometimes a general anaesthetic may be required. It's a bit like having the biopsy, but this time more skin and cells will be taken away. How much needs to be removed will depend in part on how many cells were left behind previously and how deep the melanoma has grown into the skin.

Once all the necessary cells have been removed, the area will be stitched up and left to heal.

If a particularly large area of skin has to be cut out, then a skin graft may be necessary. A thin patch of skin will be taken from a donor site elsewhere on your body, in an area where it won't show, and replaced over the area where the melanoma was. The skin from the skin graft site will be sore – a bit like a graze – for a few weeks, but the skin will grow back quite quickly.

Stages of skin cancer

If you receive your results and are told you have melanoma skin cancer, you may also receive information about the stage it's at. Doctors check to see how deep the melanoma is, as its depth affects how likely it is to spread – or already has spread – and if it might come back.

The analysis is done in conjunction with other tests you have, such as a biopsy, and the stage system helps inform you about how far the cancer has spread.

The TNM staging system is common to all cancers.

- T stands for tumour and represents the size of the tumour.

- N stands for node and indicates whether the cancer has spread to the lymph nodes.

- M stands for metastasis and is used to indicate whether the cancer has spread to another part of the body.

The second part of the staging system involves numbers; the system and grading used varies slightly between different types of cancer. In the case of skin cancer, the numbering of the stages runs from zero to four, where the lowest number represents cancer that is only in the top most layer of skin.

- Stage 0 – where the cancer is only in the top layer of the skin, or the epidermis. Sometimes this is also called carcinoma in situ.

- Stage 1 – where the cancer is less than 2cm and hasn't spread.

- Stage 2 – where the cancer is more than 2cm in size, but hasn't spread.

- Stage 3 – where the cancer has spread to tissues under the skin and may have spread to the lymph nodes as well.

- Stage 4 – where the cancer has spread to another part of the body.

The two staging systems – TNM and the numbers – can be used in conjunction with each other. So, for example, if your consultant talks about T1, this means your skin cancer tumour is small and hasn't spread.

This staging is important as it helps determine what treatment options you'll receive, but it's also a useful guideline for patients to understand what stage their skin cancer is at.

Stage 0 is the earliest stage of melanoma, which is often called pre-cancerous. The melanoma cells are only in the top layer of the skin and haven't begun to spread to any of the surrounding area. Sometimes this may be referred to as melanoma in situ. It's likely that after all of the melanoma is removed, it should be cured and you won't need any further tests.

If the melanoma is already in the deeper layers of your skin, then there's a chance the cells could have spread. If this is the case, then you'll need further tests to help determine if it has spread, and where, which will provide helpful information about what treatment you'll require.

'It's really important that people know what's normal for them so they can recognise changes that are significant and feel that they can report concerns to their GP at an early stage.'

Sara Hiom, director of health information, Cancer Research UK.

What are the treatment options?

The exact treatment you'll need depends on the stage at which your melanoma is.

With stage 1 melanomas, the first call of action is to have the mole (or area of skin) removed, which may involve a wide local excision too. You may well have had all the necessary surgical procedures done before receiving the diagnosis and, if all of the harmful cells have been taken away, you may simply require follow-up appointments.

With this stage of skin cancer, the melanoma shouldn't have spread to anywhere else in the body and the risk of spreading is low.

Again, the first part of treatment for stage 2, 3 and 4 melanomas is surgery to have the offending mole or area of skin removed, plus any tissue around the areas for cells that may still be left behind.

Stage 2 melanomas have an intermediate risk that they may come back or spread to a different part of your body after they've been removed, as they would initially have grown deeper into the skin than stage 1 melanomas.

If your skin cancer is regarded as stage 3, then it has already spread to areas such as more skin, lymph vessels or lymph glands.

Sentinel node biopsy

A new technique called sentinel node biopsy may be used to try to determine if your lymph nodes near the melanoma are affected and may be carried out in stages 2 or 3. The sentinel node is the lymph node, or group of nodes, in the area containing the cancer and they're responsible for draining tissue fluid away from the area.

The sentinel node biopsy is carried out under general or local anaesthetic. The sentinel node is found by using an injected dye (sometimes it is blue) and x-rays. The dye is injected into the area where the melanoma is and the x-ray will show the progress of the dye as it reaches the lymph nodes. The first lymph node it reaches is the sentinel node. The doctor will then remove the sentinel node and send it away to be tested.

On average, the procedure takes about 40 minutes (10 minutes for the dye to reach the sentinel node and 30 minutes for the biopsy) and is usually performed as day surgery. If you're given general anaesthetic, you may feel groggy for a while and may need pain relief as the anaesthetic wears off. It can take a while for your feeling to fully come back after a local anaesthetic. In both cases, you may have to stay resting in hospital for a while, before being allowed home. A dressing will cover the biopsy area and soluble stitches will disappear of their own accord over the next week to 10 days. If the injected dye is blue, then this will flush out through your urine, turning it green in colour; don't be alarmed, this is perfectly normal!

In cases where it's suspected that the cancer has spread away from the original site and into the lymph nodes, melanoma cells have to go through the sentinel node first in order to reach other nodes. So if the sentinel node doesn't contain cancer cells, then you won't need lymph node surgery, as it's unlikely to have spread. If cancer cells are found, then surgery will be required to remove the other nodes in the area in case they contain cancerous cells.

The lymph nodes needing to be removed depend on where the main melanoma is found and it can be quite major surgery.

Chemotherapy

Chemotherapy treatment is used to treat skin cancer that recurrs in the same place or close by, for stage 3 or 4 melanoma that has spread to another part of your body and in cases where cancer cells are found in the lymph nodes. It can also be used if the melanoma is too advanced at diagnosis for surgery to be possible.

The treatment uses special cytotoxic drugs – either one type or a combination – to destroy the cancer cells. It involves having tablets or injections for a few days, then a break of three to four weeks, followed by more treatment. Courses of chemotherapy vary in length, but you may need up to six or more cycles.

The drugs help to stop the cancer cells from growing and are designed to circulate in the blood around your body. Unfortunately, the strong nature of the drugs means that side effects are common, with sickness, diarrhoea, mouth ulcers, tiredness, hair thinning and hair loss all frequently experienced.

If you're given a combination of several drugs, then the side effects may be bad, but they should only last for the few days when you're receiving the drugs. You're also likely to get very tired towards the end of treatment courses and your energy may take a while to come back, even when the treatment has finished. If you have any side effects, then do tell your doctor or consultant, as they may be able to help.

Isolated limb perfusion

In cases where there is a secondary melanoma on your leg or arm, then a specialised procedure called isolated limb perfusion may be used. For example, it could be used for stage 3 or 4 cancer, where it has spread.

This technique uses chemotherapy drugs and allows the treatment to only be given to one limb, rather than your whole body. As less drugs are involved, this means you won't have so many side effects to the chemotherapy and shouldn't feel sick or lose any hair. It does make the treatment area sore though and you may have some pain, redness and swelling. The redness and swelling can start up to 48 hours after treatment and after the redness of your skin dies down, you can be left with a slight change of skin colour (lighter than normal).

If you could be at risk of developing a blood clot in your arm or leg, you may have to stay in hospital for a few days to be monitored.

Radiotherapy

Radiotherapy is used to treat advanced cases of melanoma in various stages, alleviate symptoms and shrink tumours. It involves using high energy rays to destroy the carcinoma and is given at the radiotherapy unit in hospital.

Radiotherapy is usually given once each day, with a break over the weekend; the cycle can be repeated for several weeks, depending on the amount of treatment you require.

Compared to chemotherapy, there are fewer side effects, though your skin in the area being treated can become sore. Depending on the part of your body being treated, some side effects can occur immediately after the treatment, but you will be advised by your doctor before the treatment starts. Although radiotherapy generally doesn't cause hair loss, it can sometimes occur in the area of the body being treated, but is usually only temporary.

It's normal to feel tired and emotional after having radiotherapy treatment and ideally you should give yourself time to rest after treatments. The exact recovery time will vary from person to person and depends on how long the course of treatment lasts.

Biological therapy

Biological therapy is sometimes used to treat some stages of melanoma; for example, to try to stop melanoma that has spread to the lymph nodes from recurring. The body naturally produces substances to help fight viral infections and one of these substances is interferon.

A special, man-made version of interferon has been produced and, with biological therapy, it's given as an injection several times a week. The idea is that it will encourage the body's immune system to help fight the cancer.

It can cause side effects, such as headaches, tiredness and fevers, which are often likened to the symptoms of flu. These are often especially prevalent when you first start the treatment, but they may lessen over time.

Future treatments

Research is continuing all the time into new treatments. Cancer vaccines are being investigated to see if they could help treat melanoma. In the future, it's hoped that vaccines for cancer will be available and could help the body's immune system to fight and destroy the cancer cells.

What if it spreads?

Melanoma can spread to anywhere else in your body, but it commonly spreads to the lungs, liver, bones, abdomen or brain.

If you have advanced stage 4 melanoma, where it's found to have spread to other parts of your body, then treatments such as chemotherapy, radiotherapy and biological therapy may all be required.

If tumours are found to have spread and appear in other parts of your body, then surgery may be required to remove them.

The exact treatment you'll have will depend on where the cancer has spread to, what treatment you've already had and the symptoms you've got. Your consultant should discuss the options with you carefully and help you decide which treatment would be best.

Checklist

- See your GP straightaway to get any suspicious moles or patches of skin checked out.

- If you are diagnosed with malignant melanoma, find out which type it is and at what stage it is.

- Don't be afraid to ask questions – your doctor is there to help.

- If you're unsure of exactly what your treatment will involve, or when it will start, ask for clarification.

'When cancers are detected earlier, treatment tends to be milder and more effective. Being generally aware of changes that could be a sign of cancer could make a crucial difference for people who do develop the disease.'

Sara Hiom, director of health information, Cancer Research UK.

Summing Up

- Malignant melanoma is the most serious form of skin cancer and can either start from a mole or an area of skin that was previously normal.

- There are four different types of malignant melanoma that affect different age groups and start in different areas of the skin – superficial spreading melanoma, nodula melanoma, lentigo maligna melanoma and acral lentiginous melanoma.

- The causes of malignant melanoma are similar to that of non-malignant melanoma, with habits such as sunbathing, using a sunbed and getting sunburnt all proving to be high risk factors.

- Spotting potential problems early on can help reduce the severity of malignant melanoma and you can use the ABCD mole rule to keep an eye out for any changes to your skin. If you do notice anything suspicious, then see your GP promptly to get it checked out.

- If malignant melanoma is suspected, a biopsy will be required to test the skin cells.

- Like other forms of cancer, the extent and severity of skin cancer is measured by the stage system. The treatment required depends in part on the stage which your melanoma is at.

- Some of the common forms of treatment include radiotherapy and chemotherapy, but new treatments are being researched.

- Malignant melanoma can spread to other parts of your body, especially if it's at an advanced stage.

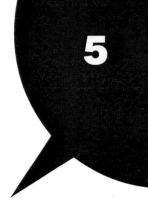

5

The Emotional Effects of Skin Cancer

earing the news that you've got skin cancer is always a shock and is likely to cause a wide range of emotional effects and reactions, both for yourself and your family and friends.

Coping with a diagnosis

No one wants to hear those words, 'You've got skin cancer,' and nothing can prepare you for receiving the diagnosis. Even though you'll already have had tests and investigations and worried about what the outcome will be, you'll no doubt have hoped, even at the back of your mind, that everything would be fine and it was all a false alarm.

It's normal to feel shocked and numb after learning the diagnosis, especially if you've otherwise been in good health. In many cases of skin cancer people only require a small amount of treatment to be successfully cured, but regardless of this, it's still a huge shock and will inevitably cause you and your immediate family to worry.

'It's normal to feel shocked and numb after learning the diagnosis, especially if you've otherwise been in good health.'

If possible, when you go to your appointments with a consultant, it's good to have someone with you, not only for support, but also so they can take in what's said or write notes for you. When you're first diagnosed, and in a state of shock, it's natural to forget or be confused about what you're told. The time you have with the consultant is often limited and there can be a lot to take in, so bringing someone along to all of your appointments, even the later ones, can be very useful.

Hearing that your skin cancer is advanced

A small minority of people will not only hear the news that they have skin cancer, but also that it's at an advanced stage and has already spread to other parts of the body.

This is understandably devastating news and extremely hard to take in. Everyone reacts in different ways and it will take time to fully comprehend what you've been told. If you feel able to share your feelings with someone else and talk about what you're going through, then having support through such a difficult time can be helpful.

Organisations such as Macmillan Cancer Support are only a phone call away, and it can really make a difference to chat with someone who understands your situation and could offer additional help and support. See the help list for their contact details.

Asking questions

With any diagnosis, it's only natural to want to ask questions so you understand your situation better. You might not have thought of them all the moment you received your diagnosis, but your consultant or specialist nurse should be available to speak to you when you've worked out what you want to ask.

Some of the key questions you may wish to ask could include:

- What stage is my skin cancer at?
- What treatment will I need and how long will it last?
- Where will the treatment be?
- What side effects are possible?
- Can I still work while having treatment?
- What is the risk of the cancer coming back?

How might I feel during treatment?

'Everyone reacts differently during treatment and it depends in part on the treatment you receive and the severity of your skin cancer.'

Everyone reacts differently during treatment and it depends in part on the treatment you receive and the severity of your skin cancer. However, some of the common feelings expressed by skin cancer patients include anger, anxiety, worry, concern and depression.

You may feel angry about developing skin cancer in the first place. 'Why me?' is a commonly expressed statement. You could be anxious about the treatment you're having and whether it will work, and worried about the possibility of the cancer coming back again. Many people are concerned about how they'll get through tough treatment regimes and still manage to keep working or maintain usual family routines for their children, and others find themselves down and depressed about the whole situation.

If you have malignant melanoma and are already having chemotherapy or radiotherapy treatment, then you may well feel tired from the treatment in addition to any other emotional feelings you have. In turn, this can affect your ability to work, get things done around the house, look after children or keep up with usual routines.

If you are experiencing depression, or any other emotional issues that are affecting your ability to cope, then do seek help or find someone to talk to. There are a variety of sources of help available, including your GP and cancer nurse. If you feel like you could gain support from talking to other people in the same situation – this can help you realise that you're not alone in what you're going through – then there may well be a cancer support group nearby, or one you can join online. The cancer helplines run by major organisations, such as Macmillan Cancer Support, can also be a great source of advice and help, whatever stage of your illness you're at.

If you are a teen or young person who is going through skin cancer, it can be a particularly isolating experience. Watching or hearing about how your friends are going out, enjoying life and being carefree can add to feelings of depression or anger at the situation you find yourself in. Specialist organisations, such as the Teenage Cancer Trust, can offer vital support for you, your family and even siblings, and there are support groups available.

However, depending on the nature of your skin cancer and whether it's easily treatable, you may find that you cope fine with it. Yes, you may be more tired than normal and need earlier nights to get more sleep, but it may not have a major impact on your lifestyle or daily routine. In essence, everyone is different.

Dealing with the effects of treatment

It doesn't really seem fair that the treatments for skin cancer can bring with them their own unpleasant side effects, but with options such as chemotherapy and radiotherapy, that's sadly often the case.

Full-blown chemotherapy is usually only used for cases of malignant melanoma, the more serious form of skin cancer. Topical chemotherapy treatment is sometimes used for non-malignant skin cancer, and doesn't bring with it the full barrage of side effects.

Chemotherapy treatment involves injections or tablets of specially designed cytotoxic drugs, which are strong enough to help prevent the cancer cells from growing. Unfortunately, their strength also means that they can make you feel rather poorly in the process, producing unwanted side effects such as sickness, hair thinning or hair loss, diarrhoea, mouth ulcers and nausea.

None of these side effects are pleasant to deal with and can make you feel really unwell. There are some remedies, such as ginger, which you can use to lessen the effects of nausea – try ginger supplements, drinking ginger tea or sucking a small piece of crystallised ginger. Over-the-counter remedies are available that can help with mouth ulcers.

Sometimes just resting and trying to relax as much as possible in between treatments will help, especially as your energy levels are likely to be depleted, and it's good to have plenty of emotional and practical support around you too.

Your changing appearance

Depending on where your skin cancer is removed from, you may feel the effects of a change in appearance. If the melanoma is removed from an area of your skin that is visible to everyone – such as your face or neck – then any scarring will be difficult to cover up.

It's normal to feel uncomfortable and upset after having skin cancer removed and it can significantly affect your confidence in your appearance if it's in an obvious place. It may take some time to get used to your new appearance, but it's important to remember that over time scars will fade and it doesn't have to change what makes you 'you'.

If you've been offered counselling, then it can help to talk through your feelings about your change in appearance and how it is affecting your life. If you don't fancy talking to a stranger, then perhaps speaking to a close friend or family member instead will help you come to terms with any loss or sadness you have about a change to your appearance.

On a practical level, even if the scarring does seem bad at first, it's often possible to successfully cover it over using clever make-up tricks. Sometimes skin clinics will offer help and advice regarding make-up and how you could cover up any areas of skin that you don't feel comfortable having on show anymore. Look Good Feel Better are a charity dedicated to helping women cancer patients – they hold free skincare and make up workshops to help improve self esteem and confidence (see help list).

Re-adjusting to life with cancer

There's no doubt that having skin cancer is likely to have an effect on your life, but how much of an impact it has will vary. It depends in part on the severity of the cancer, the treatment you're undergoing and partly on your own outlook and ability to cope with it.

If you've got non-malignant skin cancer or your cancer is at an early stage, then it may not have so much of an impact on your life and routine and you can carry on as reasonably normal.

When you're going through the stages of having treatments such as surgery, chemotherapy and radiotherapy, then it's only natural for it to have some effects. You may need to have some time off work, and you might find that you can't keep up with all your usual hobbies and evening activities, or that you need to schedule in time for a nap in the afternoon.

You may need to re-adjust your work schedule for a while or temporarily make changes to activities you're involved in. This doesn't mean long-term changes and doesn't mean you can't go back to being fully involved again soon, but while you're going through treatment for skin cancer, little changes may be needed to help you get through it all successfully.

Some people may find that they cope very well with it and the only real re-adjustment they need is in their thinking and learning to accept that they have skin cancer.

'Seeing my friend go through surgery and chemotherapy for malignant melanoma was heartbreaking. The effect of skin cancer touched us all.'

Marian.

Caring for someone with skin cancer

It can be just as hard for friends, partners or families to learn that their loved ones have skin cancer and are going to need treatment. It's common for carers to find themselves going through a barrage of emotions while trying to understand the news and take it in.

It's especially hard for those who are caring for someone with skin cancer. Treatments such as chemotherapy can cause nasty side effects and it can be difficult to see a friend or loved one in discomfort, pain and feeling unwell.

In the same way that a cancer patient may benefit from talking about what they're going through, so too can carers. Families and friends can be a good source of comfort and chat, but if, as a carer, you'd prefer talking to someone unconnected to the situation, then a counsellor could be a good option. A cancer nurse, consultant or your GP may well be able to suggest someone locally or there are national organisations, such as the British Association for Counselling and Psychotherapy, who maintain a directory of qualified counsellors (see help list).

At times it's good to be a listening ear for those being cared for, but it's also important to remember that they might not always want to discuss cancer or being ill. It can sometimes seem like skin cancer dominates life and there are times when it's more helpful to switch off and forget it, if only for a while.

For those cancer patients that have previously lived a very independent life, it can be hard to suddenly need help. It's not unusual for people to struggle on for as long as they can, even if they're having gruelling treatment, and decline offers of help.

Don't be offended if they refuse help, even if they could do with it, and instead be patient and willing to step in when they're ready.

Caring for a teenager or young person with skin cancer

Skin cancer in children is very rare, but malignant melanoma has sadly become the most common form of cancer affecting those aged 15 to 34. It can understandably be very hard for teenagers diagnosed with skin cancer to cope with it, and for those caring from them to deal with the emotions and shock that they face too.

Depending on the nature and severity of the skin cancer, the treatment regime can be exhausting for a teenager to cope with, especially if they experience side effects from the treatment.

There's also the issue of being away from friends, school, social circles or work, which can be hard to deal with – but equally difficult for their friends to deal with too.

Those caring for teenagers or young people can help by being there and listening to them when they want to talk about what they're going though – but also not pushing the issue of cancer if they don't want to discuss it.

There are various organisations that can provide help and support for both carers of teenagers and young people with cancer, and the patients themselves.

The Teenage Cancer Trust is a great source of information and advice. The charity are aware that it can be daunting and isolating for teenagers to find themselves in hospital, often with either people a lot older than themselves or younger, and are working hard to fund specialist cancer units for teenagers in NHS hospitals across the UK. Plus, the Teenage Cancer Trust also run family support networks, providing valuable support for the whole family including parents and siblings (see help list).

Finding support

Having support at hand can help you get through the low moments and difficult times of living with skin cancer. But if you don't have friends or family living close by who can give you a hand with things, or know people you can call on for extra support, then there are organisations that will be able to help.

Local support groups can put you in touch with others in similar situations and it can often be reassuring to know that you're not the only one going through certain symptoms or experiences. You could ask your consultant, GP or cancer specialist nurse if they can recommend a local support group. Macmillan Cancer Support has a searchable list of cancer support groups on their website (see help list).

Organisations such as the Cancer Counselling Trust, the British Association for Counselling and Psychotherapy and the UK Council for Psychotherapy can help put you in touch with a counsellor in your area if you need someone to talk to.

Likewise, there are organisations, such as Cruse Bereavement Care, that can offer support and help to families, friends and carers, both during a cancer experience or after the death of a loved one to cancer.

All of the organisations mentioned here, and throughout the rest of the book, are listed in the help list.

'Having support at hand can help you get through the low moments and difficult times of living with skin cancer.'

Checklist

- Ask questions if you're unsure about anything. It's good to have someone else at your appointments in case you can't remember some details.

- Investigate local support groups or organisations that may be able to help with further information, financial support or practical solutions.

- Talk to people, when you feel able to.

- Try to deal with the here and now, rather than worrying about 'what if?'

- Try to find ways to cope and adjust to the situation that work for you.

- Remember that carers need support too.

- If you need extra help, or aren't coping, seek help. There are lots of organisations offering support for cancer patients and their families.

Summing Up

- Skin cancer affects people on an emotional level as well as a physical one. Both the person with skin cancer and their family and friends can all feel the effects.

- It's only natural that being diagnosed with skin cancer can bring with it a wide array of emotions – anger, upset, shock, disbelief, worry and depression, to name but a few.

- Carers of people with skin cancer, including teenagers, young people and adults, can find it emotionally draining, but there are support groups, counsellors and cancer organisations who can provide much needed help and advice.

- Cancer shouldn't be something you go through alone and support is often available from family, friends or your local community.

- Support groups can help you feel less isolated and that you're not the only ones coping with this dreadful disease.

- Some forms of treatment for skin cancer, such as surgery, radiotherapy and chemotherapy, bring with them their own side effects and changes which can be hard to deal with too.

- Everyone re-adjusts to life with skin cancer differently. If your cancer is at an early stage, or not so serious, then it may not have such a major impact on your life as those coping with malignant melanoma.

6

Life After Skin Cancer

Many cases of skin cancer are effectively treated and cured, but everyone is different and it can take a while to get back to normality or adjust to life after skin cancer.

Common feelings that can remain for a while are those of anxiety, sadness or worry. It can take a while to get over or accept all that you've been through, especially if you've had extensive treatment or life-changing surgery, and it's normal to feel worried or anxious that the cancer might return.

Can malignant and non-malignant melanoma reccur?

'Being clued up about sun safety is even more important once you've had skin cancer. Doctors advise against exposing unprotected skin to strong sunlight.'

If you've had malignant or non-malignant melanoma in the past, then you may have a higher than average risk of getting it again in years to come. New skin cancers can occur close to or at the same site as the original skin cancer, or on areas of the skin that have been exposed to radiotherapy treatment.

It's also possible for new cases of skin cancer to appear on a completely different part of your body. No one wants to experience skin cancer twice, so it's important to be vigilant by getting into the habit of regularly checking your skin and adapting your lifestyle to look after your skin to the best of your ability.

Being clued up about sun safety is even more important once you've had skin cancer. Doctors advise against exposing unprotected skin to strong sunlight.

This doesn't mean that you can't enjoy being outside or going on holiday to sunny climes – far from it – but you will need to be sensible and take the necessary precautions to help protect your skin.

This includes following the basic sun safety measures, such as using an SPF15+ broad-spectrum sunscreen, staying out of the sun between 11am and 3pm, and wearing a hat, sunglasses and cotton clothing with a tight weave when you're outdoors in the summer. A broad-spectrum sunscreen is a product that offers protection against both UVA and UVB rays. The amount of UVB protection is measured by the SPF and the amount of UVA protection by the UVA star system.

Getting into the habit of checking your skin

After you've had either malignant or non-malignant skin cancer, then it is important to get into the habit of regularly checking your skin and knowing what's normal and what's not. For areas that you can't see so easily yourself, such as on your back, then it's useful to get a friend or partner that you trust to check for you.

According to the NICE guidelines, if you've had a skin cancer that has a lower risk of recurring, then you should be taught self-examination techniques by your GP, specialist or cancer nurse and given advice about what to look out for. If for any reason you're unable to self-examine, then medical professionals should provide some other way for your condition to be monitored.

If you've had skin cancer and have a higher risk of it reccurring, you should also be taught self-examination techniques. The NICE guidelines also suggest that people should be given both written information about what to look for as well as photographs to help with self-examinations.

As a rule of thumb, try to get into the routine of checking every two months for any changes or unusual patches that appear on your skin and don't heal or go away within four to six weeks. For example:

- A spot or sore patch of skin that appears and doesn't heal within a month.

- A spot or sore area of skin that itches, is painful, crusted over or bleeds continuously for a month.

- Skin that has formed into an ulcer for no apparent reason and doesn't heal within a month.

If you notice any changes or new developments that concern you, then you should report it to your GP or your skin cancer specialist or cancer nurse, if you're still under their care.

> 'Try to get into the routine of checking your skin every two months for any changes or unusual patches that appear on your skin and don't heal or go away within four to six weeks.'

Are there long-term effects of skin cancer?

When you've recently finished treatment for skin cancer, it's normal to feel tired and have lower energy levels than usual, which can go on for months or even a year after your treatment, but over time this should gradually improve.

Likewise, although you may be physically better, the effect of having had skin cancer can have an impact and may leave you feeling anxious, concerned, depressed or upset about it for a while. If you find yourself in this situation, then it may well help to get yourself some extra support, either from talking to friends or family, speaking to a GP or cancer nurse, or a skin cancer support group. It can be reassuring to learn that you're not the only one left reeling from the shock of having had skin cancer.

If you're feeling very depressed, then you should see your GP, as you may benefit from either talking about your worries with a professional counsellor or from an anti-depressant prescription to help you through the worst.

Post-cancer skin strategy

One of the long-term issues to be aware of is that, as a result of having had skin cancer once, you'll subsequently be at a higher than average risk of getting it again. Due to this, it's even more important that you take care of your skin, especially when outside, and that you should completely avoid using a sunbed.

As a general rule of thumb, if you've had skin cancer, you should be clued up on the safe sun guidelines and:

- Get into the habit of wearing close weave cotton clothing when out and about on sunny days.

- Opt for long sleeves and trousers, rather than shorts.

- Choose to wear a hat that offers good protection for your face and neck.

- Avoid being out in the sun when it's at its strongest, from 11am to 3pm.

- Always use broad-spectrum sunscreen and opt for a high factor. The highest factor sunscreen is factor 60 which will filter out about 98% of the harmful rays.

- Wear the wraparound style of sunglasses to add protection for your eyes.

- Never allow your skin to get burnt.

Life insurance and travel insurance

After you've had skin cancer, it can become more difficult or more expensive to get travel insurance or life insurance. It's frustrating, especially when your skin cancer has been successfully treated and you're feeling well enough to go and have a holiday.

Even though you may find that your usual insurance company is now too expensive for you to use, it's worth checking around and getting quotes from other companies. There are some insurance companies, for example, who are more geared up to insuring people with existing or past health problems and they may well consider insuring cancer patients.

Over time, and assuming you don't have any recurrences of the cancer, then it should in theory become easier to obtain insurance, and the cost of your insurance premiums should go down.

The importance of regular check-ups

As well as doing your own self checks to make sure your skin is looking okay, you may well have to have regular check-ups and follow-up appointments with your consultant too.

NICE guidelines set out recommendations for follow-up care. In the case of skin cancer, these depend in part on the type of skin cancer you've had, the level of risk involved, the treatment you had and where the skin cancer was located. Your follow-up care should be jointly agreed by your doctor or consultant and yourself, and you should be given individual guidance about how often to expect follow-ups.

In some cases, if everything has gone well, it was a routine removal of skin cancer and your treatment has been successful, then you could be discharged from the care of your consultant quite quickly. If you've had a lower risk form of skin cancer, then follow-up care may be offered at a treatment centre, community hospital or via your GP.

If you're deemed to be at a higher risk of getting skin cancer again then you may need to be monitored on a more ongoing basis by specialists at the hospital.

Regaining your life after skin cancer

Like any other form of cancer, having skin cancer can have a major effect on your life. Although you may feel relieved that your treatment is finally over, it's not always easy to immediately pick up the pieces and go back to how you were before your cancer experience. Some people do seem to effortlessly manage it, but for others, there's still a lot of adjusting to do and it takes time to work through the emotional issues and come to terms with everything.

It's not always easy to put the pain, discomfort and worry of skin cancer behind you, and some people always have the fear that it will return at the back of their mind, but trying to get back to some degree of normality is an important part of the post-cancer recovery process.

Marking the end of treatment

Some people find that marking the end of treatment and the recovery period can be a good way of signifying that that part of their cancer experience is now over. Plus, it can give you something to look forward to, focus on and aid positivity as you go through the final stages of recovery.

For example, going on a long-awaited holiday, even if it doesn't involve travelling all that far, is a popular choice, or you might like to treat yourself to something special or get your house redecorated. It doesn't matter what you choose to do, but doing something to mark the occasion can be very therapeutic.

Regaining your routine

When it comes to re-adjusting and regaining your life on a more permanent basis, some people feel fine about picking things up where they left off and carrying on the same job or routine as in their pre-cancer days.

But there's always the possibility that you might not want to go back to exactly how things were before – some people find they have had time to reflect or decide they want to make changes to their life after going through cancer.

For example, this could be changes to your lifestyle, like giving up sunbathing or tanning, which can be a big change if you've previously been a sun or tanning devotee. Or it could be something like changes to your diet, such as eating healthier or exercising more, or using your spare time differently and getting involved in new challenges or hobbies.

'I had non-malignant skin cancer on my arm. It was a shock to hear the news, but I'm thankful the treatment was successful and I got through it okay.'

Greg.

Whether you're planning to celebrate the end of your treatment, want to make changes to your previous lifestyle or to get back to normal as soon as possible, then you're free to do so in the way you feel is best for you.

Checklist

- Make sure you're confident with self-examining your skin – your GP or specialist should show you how.

- Be sure to adopt a safe sun strategy to limit any further damage to your skin.

- Check with your GP or specialist about follow-up appointments and check-ups.

- Shop around for life insurance and travel insurance if you need new policies.

- If you feel you'd like to, mark the end of your treatment with a celebration or treat.

- Don't worry if you don't want to pick up life exactly where you left it – a new routine may do you the world of good.

Summing Up

- Skin cancer can be successfully treated, but having a serious disease can have a major impact on your life.

- There is often the worry that malignant or non-malignant skin cancer could reccur, as people who've had skin cancer may be left with a higher risk of getting it again.

- To protect your skin and reduce the risk of more skin cancer, it's advisable to avoid exposing your skin to strong sunlight, as well as wearing a high factor, broad-spectrum sunscreen and following sun safety guidelines.

- If you've had skin cancer, it's important to get firmly into the habit of regularly checking your skin. Your GP or specialist may teach self-examination techniques, but otherwise it's useful to self-examine skin every two months.

- Many people feel tired and have lower energy levels after treatment for skin cancer and the experience of going through it all can leave people feeling anxious, depressed or upset for a while.

- Adopting a post-cancer sun strategy can help reduce the risk of developing skin cancer again.

- People who've had skin cancer, and other forms of cancer, often find that it's more expensive or difficult to subsequently obtain travel insurance. Although it can be frustrating finding a suitable insurer, shopping around and getting different quotes can eventually lead to a more cancer-friendly insurance provider.

- Regular check-ups with your GP or consultant may be necessary. The NICE guidelines set out recommendations for follow-up care. Your care programme should be agreed jointly by your GP, consultant and yourself.

- Some people can't wait to get back to their old routine after skin cancer, while other people are keen to make changes to their lives. You should do whatever you feel comfortable doing.

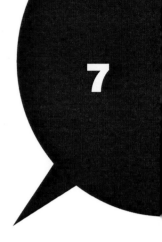

7

All About Sunscreen

One of the vital ways in which we can learn to protect our skin and help reduce the risk of developing skin cancer is through regular use of sunscreen. It's readily available, but do you know which SPF factor is best for your skin, how often to use it or how much to apply?

Does sunscreen really work?

'The main factors to look out for are the SPF – sun protection factor – and the broad-spectrum star rating of a sunscreen product. These two elements are indicators of how much protection the sunscreens offer.'

Sunscreen is a special product that's been developed to help protect the skin from UVA and UVB rays. If you're going to be spending time outside in the sun, even if it's only for short periods of time, then it's well worth investing in sunscreen to help protect your skin.

Although no sunscreen offers total protection against UVA and UVB rays, it's a great help to use in the fight against skin cancer and is one of the practical ways in which you can protect your skin.

Studies into sunscreen have shown that sunscreen can protect against the effects of UV radiation, and one study into broad-spectrum sunscreen indicated that people who use sunscreens have less moles than those who don't. As moles are a big risk factor for malignant melanomas, this is an encouraging finding.

Sunscreen isn't the only form of protection needed though, and it's best used in conjunction with other methods, such as staying out of the hot midday sun, covering up by wearing a hat, sunglasses and a loose t-shirt, and not letting your skin burn.

Just because you've put sunscreen on, this doesn't mean it's an excuse to stay out longer or that your skin won't burn. It's still important to play it safe in the sun, whether you're wearing sunscreen or not, and it's especially important to keep a close eye on children's skin, as their skin can burn far more quickly.

Which SPF sunscreen to choose

There are so many different sunscreens on the market that it's often overwhelming and hard to know what to choose. Although there are lots of different brands and prices, the main factors to look out for are the SPF – sun protection factor – and the broad-spectrum star rating of a product. These two elements are indicators of how much protection the sunscreens offer.

SPF system

The SPF of a sunscreen tells you how much protection the sunscreen offers against the sun's UVB rays – the ones that cause sunburn and skin cancer. The higher the SPF factor, the more protection you gain against burning, but not necessarily against UVA radiation.

Although it's easy to assume that if you choose a sunscreen with an SPF of 30 you must be getting double the protection of an SPF15, this is sadly not the case. An SPF15 will filter out 93% of UVB radiation, whereas an SPF30 will filter out 96%. This is 3% more protection, not 50%, as some people assume. Even an SPF60, which is the highest factor sunscreen, only filters out 98% of the sun's rays – or a mere 5% more than SPF15. For most people, an SPF15 sunscreen is sufficient.

The SPF is determined by measuring how long skin covered with sunscreen takes to burn, compared to uncovered skin. For example, an SPF of 30 means it will take 30 minutes longer to burn when wearing the sunscreen. Whatever the SPF of your sunscreen, you should aim to reapply it regularly throughout the day if you're outside and exposed to sunlight. Choosing a higher SPF should not be used as an excuse to only apply it once a day or stay out in the sun longer.

Choosing which SPF to go for depends in part on your skin type – how pale it is and how easily you burn. If you have very pale or fair skin, light or red hair, and skin that either burns easily or often, then you're better off with a high-factor sunscreen.

Cancer experts suggest that an SPF15 sunscreen is appropriate for the average person in Europe and should provide enough protection from even the hottest midday summer sun.

UVA star system

The amount of UVA protection offered by a broad-spectrum sunscreen is shown using a star rating system, which runs from zero stars (no protection) to five stars (the best). If a product has a five UVA star rating, then it should have roughly the same amount of protection against UVA rays as it has against UVB rays.

With products that have less than a five star UVA rating, then you'll be getting less UVA than UVB protection. If you want your skin to get the maximum protection available, than you should aim to choose a sunscreen with a high SPF and four to five UVA stars.

Organic versus inorganic sunscreens

Two other bits of terminology that you may come across in relation to sunscreens are organic and inorganic. Forget the usual meaning of organic, as in sunscreen terms it doesn't mean that it's natural.

Instead, organic (or chemical) suncreens work like sponges, by absorbing the UV light on the surface of your skin, which stops the light getting in.

Inorganic (or mineral) sunscreens work like mirrors, by reflecting the light away from the surface of the skin before it can get in.

Many brands of sunscreen are now a mix of both organic and inorganic.

How much sunscreen to use

Once you've purchased your bottle of sunscreen, how much do you have to use each time to get the benefit of its protection?

One of the biggest mistakes made by users of sunscreen is not applying enough and not reapplying later in the day. It's all very well investing in a high factor sunscreen, but not much use if you don't apply enough of it, as you won't gain the crucial benefits. Just because it's a higher-factor sunscreen doesn't mean you can apply less of it than a lower-factor sunscreen!

If you're looking to apply sunscreen to your arms, neck and face, then you need to allow approximately two teaspoonfuls of sunscreen.

If you want to cover your entire body with sunscreen, for example if you're on a beach, or working in a job where you're fully out in the sun and your skin is exposed, then you should aim to put on two tablespoonfuls of sunscreen in each application.

How to apply sunscreen

Apply the sunscreen to clean, dry skin – ideally, before you put on any moisturiser, skin care products or cosmetics – and before you go out in the sun.

You should apply an ample amount of sunscreen to all areas of the skin that will be exposed. Don't forget areas that could be vulnerable, such as your feet, hands, neck and even your ears.

'UV rays are invisible and can't be felt on the skin, but can damage skin cells leading to sunburn and an increased risk of skin cancer. So even if it's a breezy summer day when it may not feel as warm, the potential for sunburn is still there.'

Sara Hiom, director of health information, Cancer Research UK.

How often to apply sunscreen

Ideally, sunscreen should be applied to your skin first thing in the morning, or 15 to 30 minutes before you go outside. It can help to make it a habit to apply it at a certain time – e.g. make it part of your morning routine to put it on before you put your makeup on, or before you get dressed.

If you're out and about a lot, then sunscreen should be reapplied every two hours, or more often if you're on holiday and in and out of the water.

Even though some types of sunscreen are marketed with the message that they only need to be applied once a day, to get the best possible protection, reapplying throughout the day is still recommended.

Children and sunscreen

With their delicate, vulnerable skin, it's essential that children should be protected from the harmful effects of the sun by wearing sunscreen.

It's not just during holiday time that sunscreen should be applied – ideally, it should form part of the daily routine from April to September, and especially during the hot summer months.

Parents can help ensure sunscreen is applied before children head off to school, but as the effects wear off during the day, a reapplication is required.

For schoolchildren, it's ideal if they can apply sunscreen before they go out in the sun at break time or lunchtime, especially as lunchtime breaks often coincide with the midday sun, when the sun is at its hottest.

If your child has ever suffered an allergic reaction to a sunscreen, then Cancer Research UK suggests that inorganic sunscreens may be a better choice. This is because they're not absorbed into the skin quite so much. The ingredients of inorganic chemicals to look out for include 'titanium dioxide' and 'zinc oxide'.

There are some sunscreens particularly marketed at babies and children, which you may want to use, especially for very young children. One of the major benefits is that they're less likely to contain fragrances or other ingredients that may irritate delicate skin and are a good option if your child suffers from any known allergic reactions.

'If you're looking to apply sunscreen to your arms, neck and face, then you need to allow approximately two teaspoonfuls of sunscreen.'

Water and sunscreen

If you're going to be swimming, such as at the beach or in an outdoor swimming pool, then you'll still need to apply sunscreen to protect your skin from the effects of the sun.

If you use normal sunscreen, then it will simply wash off when you get in the water. To help combat this, there are a variety of specially produced water resistant sunscreen products available that offer full protection when you're in water.

When you're intending on going swimming – or even if you might go near the water – always apply your water-resistant sunscreen before you get in the water. Like standard sunscreen, ideally you should use a generous amount and apply it to the whole of your body. If you're frequently getting in and out of the water, then reapply the sunscreen regularly.

Be aware that some sunscreens are designed to be sweatproof, but this is different to waterproof, so make sure you get the right one for your needs. Whereas waterproof sunscreens are designed to have water on the outside of the skin, the sweatproof sunscreens cater for sweat that forms on the inside of the skin.

The importance of sunscreen on cloudy days

It's often assumed that you only need to apply sunscreen on hot, sunny days, but it's important on cloudy days too.

In the UK, we should be thinking about sun protection issues from April to September. In general, the UV radiation is at its peak during the summer months from 11am to 3pm daily.

Even when the sun isn't shining and it's an overcast, cloudy day, up to 30% or 40% of UV can still get through the cloud and reach our skin.

It's not only cloud that can be penetrated by UV rays – the same goes for glass. Although most glass will be able to block out UVB rays, it doesn't stop the UVA rays. So if you're sitting in a car, or by a window during the summer, you can still be exposed to the harmful effects of the sun.

Winter suncare

Sun protection is important during the winter too, particularly if you're indulging in skiing or snowboarding.

The snow can reflect up to 85% of the UV radiation, even on cloudy days, and it can increase your exposure. In fact, research into the effects of UV radiation in the Alps has shown that skiers and snowboarders who spend time enjoying skiing activities at high altitudes can increase their UV exposure by up to 15% per 1,000 metres height.

How long does sunscreen last before going off?

All sunscreens should have a use-by date printed on them so you know how long they'll last before going off. As a rough idea, most will last for two to three years after opening, but for a more accurate guide, look out for the little logo on the back of sunscreen bottles that will tell you how long a product lasts after it's been opened.

It looks like a little bottle or pot symbol and will have a number printed on it, such as 12m or 18m (see below). This lets you know that, after opening, the product will last for 12 months (12m) or 18 months (18m). The symbol appears on a wide range of skincare and cosmetic products and is a useful guideline to follow, as long as you remember vaguely when you bought and opened the product.

To help preserve the life of your sunscreen it's best stored in a cool, dry place, such as a cupboard.

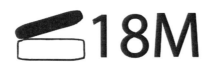

Aftersun lotions – are they any use?

As well as sunscreens, there are lots of products available that are marketed as aftersun lotions. But do you really need to fork out on buying these too?

The idea of aftersun lotions is that they're specially made to be used when you've gone back inside after being out in the sun. It's not just a product with a fancy name – they do serve a purpose and the products are carefully formulated for use after sun exposure.

For example, they have high levels of cooling ingredients in them which help to cool, calm and remoisturise the skin. You don't necessarily need to use them, but if you feel like your skin could do with cooling and calming, then it is an available option and they could be beneficial.

Checklist

- Choose a broad-spectrum sunscreen for UVB and UVA protection.
- Get clued up about how much sunscreen to use.
- Remember to put sunscreen on before you go out.
- Don't forget to reapply sunscreen.
- Encourage children to wear sunscreen from April to September, reapplying throughout the day.
- Choose waterproof sunscreen if you're going to be in water.
- Throw away any sunscreens that are past their use-by date or have been stored incorrectly.
- Don't forget that UV radiation can get through cloud too.

Summing Up

- Sunscreen is a specially developed skincare product that can be used by anyone to help protect their skin from the harmful effects of the sun's rays.

- No sunscreen will offer 100% protection, but they can make a significant difference, especially if used in conjunction with other sun safety measures, such as wearing a hat, sunglasses and loose clothing.

- The SPF of a sunscreen stands for the sun protection factor. This tells you how much protection the sunscreen offers against the sun's UVB rays.

- A broad-spectrum sunscreen also offers protection against UVA. The UVA star system indicates how much protection is offered.

- Organic sunscreens work by absorbing the UV light like a sponge, whereas inorganic sunscreens work by reflecting the light, like a mirror.

- Ideally, you should apply two teaspoonfuls of sunscreen in each application, to your arms, neck and face. If applying sunscreen to your whole body, allow for two tablespoons of sunscreen per application.

- Sunscreen should be applied 15 to 30 minutes before you go outside and children should have some on before going to school. If you're on a beach or in and out of a pool, be aware that normal sunscreen will wash off. So opt for a water-resistant sunscreen instead.

- Even when the sun isn't shining, UV radiation can get through, so continue to apply sunscreen on cloudy days. It's also an issue in the winter, as snow can reflect UV radiation and increase your exposure.

- On average, sunscreen will last two to three years before going off, as long as it's kept in a cool, dry place. If you're unsure, look for the symbol on the bottle to see how long it will last.

- Aftersun lotions are designed to be used after sunscreens and can cool, calm and remoisturise the skin after sun exposure.

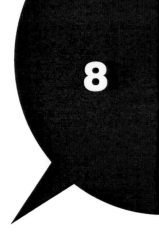

Skin Cancer Prevention

The risk of developing skin cancer can be prevented by taking care in the sun. As well as wearing sunscreen, there are plenty of other practical methods that can be put into action, whether you're a parent looking after a baby, a child at school, or working in a job that entails being outside in the heat of the sun.

Developing safe sun habits

It's important for everyone to think about developing safe sun habits and it's never too late to do so. Whatever your age, there's still a risk of developing skin cancer if your skin is frequently exposed to UV radiation or you get sunburnt a lot.

Sometimes adults may be a bit blasé about skin protection. Their views may stem from previous ignorance about the dangers of sunbathing, or a time when less was known about the effects of UV radiation.

'It's important for everyone to think about developing safe sun habits and it's never too late to do so.'

But even if you've been lucky enough not to be affected by skin cancer in your life so far, this doesn't mean you'll never get it. In fact, UV radiation exposure builds up over time and a number of forms of skin cancer are more prevalent in middle-aged and older people, so really everyone should be taking note and taking action.

Safe sun habits are really not a hassle to remember or implement. If you can reduce the risk of developing a potentially deadly disease by simply putting some sunscreen on your skin, moving into the shade at the hottest times of the day, wearing a sun hat or covering up exposed areas of your skin, then surely it's worth the effort?

Teaching children about sun safety

It's important for everyone to learn about sun safety habits and that includes children, especially as about 80% of our sun exposure is gained by the time we're 21 years old. Although it's rare for young children to get skin cancer, for teens aged 15 and over, melanoma is the most common cancer for their age group.

Children's skin is more delicate than adults' and it's even more prone to sun damage. This damage is stored up and can develop into skin cancer at a later stage, but by reducing the amount of sun exposure and sunburn, this risk can be significantly reduced.

This doesn't mean children can't spend time outside – just that it's better to do so while taking a few extra precautions. If children are used to safe sun habits, then hopefully they'll continue practising them long into the future.

The key sun safety messages

The key sun safety messages to pass on to children are:

- Stay out of the sun when it's at its hottest, from about 11am until 3pm. If you have to be outside during those times, then stay in the shade.

- Wear sunscreen to protect your skin and to get into the habit of putting it on before you go out.

- Clothing is a good way of covering up and protecting your skin.

- Wear a hat to protect your head, and sunglasses to protect the eyes.

- Reapply sunscreen if you've been in water.

- Sunscreen and hats aren't just something to think about at home, they're also important at school too.

Sun safety in schools

As more has become known about the dangers of the sun and as skin cancer cases have increased, schools have, in general, become more clued up about sun dangers. In fact, many schools are doing well with their sun safety measures.

The typical timings of school break times and lunchtimes mean that many children are outside in the summer months when the sun is at its peak. The sun safety message suggests that it's best to stay in the shade from 11am to 3pm, but school playgrounds may not be the shadiest of places.

Thankfully, more is being done now to ensure that shady areas are available in school grounds, through trees, canopies, shelters, sun umbrellas or even buildings. The Cancer Research UK SunSmart campaign has played an important part in helping schools realise the importance of sun safety and suggests ideas for how more shade can be achieved.

'Avoiding excessive exposure to UV can dramatically reduce a person's risk of developing skin cancer.'

Sara Hiom, director of health information, Cancer Research UK.

In addition to staying in the shade, other useful sun protection methods that can be encouraged by schools include the use of sunscreen and wearing hats. Even if sunscreen has been put on first thing in the morning, perhaps before going to school, by the time lunchtime arrives, a reapplication would be required.

Some schools are happy for sunscreen to be supplied by parents and then put on by children before they go out in the playground. In the case of younger children, such as infants or nursery age, then teachers may need to assist in the task.

Another simple way of reducing the risk, whether there is shade provided or not, is to wear a hat or cap outside during lunchtime and breaks. The most protective hat is one that covers the head, face, neck and ears.

Keeping babies safe in the sun

As chapter 2 discussed, babies are particularly at risk from the effects of the sun, as they have very delicate and thin skin which is easily damaged. Even being burnt badly once during childhood is linked to an increased risk of skin cancer later in life.

Due to this, it's essential that parents do all they can to protect vulnerable babies when they're out and about in the sun. This doesn't mean that you can't spend time outside when the sun is shining – far from it – but that a few precautions can make the experience better for everyone.

If you're out walking with your baby in a pram or buggy, then ensure they have sufficient shade from the full glare of the sun. Choose places to sit outside that benefit from plenty of shade, such as under trees, sun umbrellas or canopies, and be aware that as the sun moves, it may encroach on your shade, requiring you to adjust position.

Babies can be covered up well with loose-fitting clothes and, although they may not be keen on wearing a hat, do try to encourage it. A wide-brimmed hat is ideal, as it covers their face, ears and neck.

When you're buying sunscreen, look out for products that are specially designed for babies. Although you can use ordinary sunscreens too, the products aimed at babies are less likely to contain ingredients that may irritate delicate skin or cause allergic reactions.

Sun safety at work

For people in some areas of employment, such as builders, traffic wardens, lifeguards, gardeners or farmers, the very nature of their job means that they're outside a lot of the time. In an ideal world, it would be possible to avoid having to work during the hottest time of the day, but sadly in many cases that isn't possible, so workers invariably end up outside in the full force of the sun.

Research has shown that outdoor workers who spend much or all of their working time outside have an average of three to four times more exposure to harmful UV each year than people who work indoors. People who have fair skin in particular, who are already at risk of sunburn and skin cancer, will find themselves in a less than ideal situation if they do outdoor jobs.

This is not helped by the fact that when it gets very hot, it's only natural to want to try to cool down by wearing thinner clothes, short sleeves or shorts, but this gives skin even more exposure. Men who work outside without a shirt on really are putting their skin at risk.

According to the Health and Safety at Work Act (1974) and the Management of Health and Safety at Work Regulations (1999), all employers have a legal duty to protect the health and safety of their employees and this applies to sun safety issues too.

Ideally, employers should offer solutions to help workers avoid too much exposure to the midday sun, encourage them to adopt sun safety procedures, such as covering up, and consider offering them sunscreen.

For example, outdoor tasks could be adapted to be performed at times of the day when the sun isn't so hot (earlier or later) or staff could be rotated so that no one is in the midday heat for an extensive period. Where possible, shade could be provided or hats could be added to the uniform to offer a bit of extra protection.

If sun safety at work is a concern to you, either as an employee or an employer, and you want to try to improve the help available, then Cancer Research UK have a free factsheet available entitled 'SunSmart Strategies for the Workplace'. See www.sunsmart.org.uk for more details.

'Outdoor workers who spend much or all of their working time outside have an average of three to four times more exposure to harmful UV each year.'

What to wear to protect yourself

Although it may seem natural to want to wear less clothing when it's really hot outside, in order to protect your skin, taking care with what you wear and covering up can help. This is especially the case if there isn't any shade available.

Clothing made from materials with a close weave will help block out most of the UV rays. If you're not sure if it's a close weave material, then try holding the item of clothing up to the light and see how much light can get through – if it doesn't allow much light, then it's a good, close weave.

If you're on a beach or near a pool, then be aware that the protection of clothing, particularly of cotton, can be affected by water. For example, a wet item of clothing, such as a shirt, may offer less protection than a dry shirt.

Hats, especially wide-brimmed varieties, are an excellent way of keeping your head, face, neck and ears protected – and with such a wide array of hats available these days, you can choose something to match your taste!

Sunglasses, too, are a big fashion statement and they help protect your eyes. To get the most protection from sunglasses, look out for products that have a 'UV 400' label and specifically say that they offer 100% UV protection. It's also advisable to look out for the CE Mark on them and the British Standard BS EN 1836:1997. Sunglasses that wrap around the side of the face will offer the maximum protection.

Checklist

- Think about your sun habits – are they safe?
- Does your child's school have a sun safety strategy? If not, why not suggest it's given some thought.
- Remember to keep babies safe in the sun, as they're particularly vulnerable.
- If you're worried about sun safety at work, speak to your employer and encourage them to adopt safe sun strategies.
- Think about your clothing – is it giving you the best sun protection?
- Invest in wraparound sunglasses to protect your face and eyes.

Summing Up

- Cases of skin cancer can be prevented by increased awareness and especially by adopting practical sun safety measures.

- It's never too late to adopt safe sun habits and is something that all ages, young or old, should think about doing.

- Adults can help spread the word about being safe in the sun by teaching children sun safety measures. This is especially important as nearly 80% of our sun exposure is gained by the time we're 21 years old and sun damage builds up over the years.

- Some of the key sun safety measures to pass on to children include the benefit of wearing sunscreen, covering up with clothes, wearing a hat to protect the head and staying out of the sun between 11am and 3pm, when it's at its hottest.

- Sun safety is important at both home and school, especially as children are often outside in the playground on their lunch break during the peak sun time.

- Babies have very vulnerable skin and need to be given plenty of protection from the harsh UV light of the sun. They can be helped by providing shade in prams and buggies, wearing sunscreen and a hat.

- People who work outdoors are exposed to three to four times more UV each year than those in indoor jobs. Ideally employers should take note of health and safety regulations and provide outdoor workers with suitable sun safety measures.

- For anyone, clothing is a good means of protecting your skin, even when it's hot. Choose clothes made from a close weave that will block out UV rays and opt for sunglasses that offer added UV protection.

9

Sunbeds and Tanning

Sunbeds are still widely available in the UK, but they are a major risk factor in the development of skin cancer. There's also still a lot of emphasis in some circles on the idea that having a tan is healthy, but is that really the case? And is there a safer method?

'Not only are sunbeds now classified in the highest risk category for cancer alongside tobacco, but there's also strong scientific evidence to show the damage they cause to the skin – both increasing skin cancer risk and ageing the skin.'

Sarah Woolnough, head of policy, Cancer Research UK.

Can using a sunbed cause skin cancer?

Sunbeds are often promoted as a good way to 'top up' or get a tan, but they are not a safe alternative to sunbathing outdoors. In fact, they can be just as dangerous as lying outside in the sun and are a major risk factor for cancer.

In the same way that the sun emits harmful UV rays, so too do sunbeds. In fact, in some cases the UV rays from sunbeds can be 10 to 15 times stronger than that of the midday sun, which can badly affect the skin.

The effect of the UV hitting and penetrating the skin can damage the DNA of skin cells, which in turn can cause premature ageing and the development of skin cancer. By premature ageing, it not only means the chance of getting wrinkles at an earlier age, but that your skin is likely to become coarse and leathery too.

The harmful effects of UV builds up over time, and every single time you lie back under a sunbed, you're damaging your skin. Statistics from Cancer Research UK suggest that if you use a sunbed before the age of 35, you increase your risk of developing melanoma skin cancer by 75%.

Anyone that uses a sunbed on a regular basis, such as once a month or more, is increasing their risk of skin cancer by at least 50%.

Who shouldn't use a sunbed?

Ideally, no one should use a sunbed but, as is the case with sunbathing, there are some groups of people that are at even more risk of developing skin cancer if they use a sunbed. Due to these increased risks, you should avoid using a sunbed if:

- You have very fair or freckled skin.
- You know that your skin burns easily.
- You have a lot of moles.
- You have a family history of skin cancer.
- You're under 18 years old.

- You're pregnant.
- You're taking any medication that can increase your sensitivity to UV light.
- You've had skin cancer already.

Aren't short sunbed sessions okay?

Even though sunbed sessions are often short, this doesn't mean they're less harmful. Lying on a sunbed for a short time, receiving intense exposure to UV light, is the easiest and quickest way to cause damage to your skin. Neither is it safe or recommended to try to increase your tan by having two or more sunbed sessions in close proximity to each other, such as within 24 hours.

Put simply, although sunbeds may be promoted and marketed as being a good way to get a tan, they're not. In reality, they're a good way to get skin cancer.

Sunbed safety

With everything we now know about the dangers of sunbeds, it seems astonishing that the practice of using a sunbed is still going on and that it's unregulated in many places.

Tanning salons first began to appear in about the 1980s, with home tanning devices also being used by some people, but they've grown in number over the last 10 years and can now be found on many a high street, with about 5,000-6,000 tanning salons in the UK.

Sadly, it also still seems to be a popular habit for some young people, who use sunbeds to try to get rid of their pale skin and get a tan. It's not helped by the fact that some tanning salons are unstaffed and have coin operated machines, which can be used again and again. There have been frequent cases reported in the media of young people using sunbeds too frequently and for too long at a time and suffering from dreadful burning as a result.

In November 2009, Scotland took the worthwhile step of banning under 18s from using sunbeds. Campaigners in Scotland, which include Cancer Research UK, are also hoping to raise awareness of the risks and ensure all adults that use sunbeds are fully aware of the facts.

'Using sunbeds has no general health benefits. In fact the intensity of UV rays in some sunbeds can be more than 10 times stronger than the midday sun and damage from UV builds up over time. So whenever people use a sunbed they are harming their skin and increasing their risk of skin cancer.'

Sarah Woolnough, head of policy, Cancer Research UK.

Although sunbed use is not recommended at all for under 18s in the rest of the UK, studies have shown that the recommendations are frequently ignored. Even in cases where tanning salons do display notices that the sunbeds shouldn't be used by under 18s (members of The Sunbed Association are advised to ban under 16s), they don't always check the ages of young people booking slots or using the equipment, which defeats the object.

A survey carried out by Cancer Research UK, for example, revealed that half of all 15 to 17 year old girls in Sunderland and Liverpool were regular users of sunbeds – with 40% using them at least once a week. A year before, in 2008, a survey by *Which?* magazine found that about 170,000 under 16 year olds in the UK had used a sunbed – a worryingly high number.

Is tanning ever safe?

Despite the dangers we now know about the sun and sunbeds, there's still a misconception that having a tan is somehow connected to looking healthy. Neither sunbathing nor using sunbeds is recommended, as both have a strong link with the risk of skin cancer, so tanning via either method is certainly not safe.

The darkening of the skin that occurs after being out in the sun is produced when UV rays trigger the production of the pigment melanin in the skin. This process produces what we know as a tan.

Ironically, far from being healthy, this is in fact a sign that the skin has been damaged and is trying to protect itself. Even if you haven't been burnt, the skin has still been damaged and continued exposure can increase the risk of skin cancer, as well as cause premature ageing. The tan may fade over time, but the damage to your skin will remain.

Likewise, sunbeds may be promoted as a way of getting a tan, but the UV light that they emit can seriously damage the skin and increase the risk of skin cancer, so it's definitely not a safe activity.

If you've read the facts and still crave a tanned-skin look, then the only truly safe way of tanning is to use fake tan, out of a bottle. Thankfully there are plenty of fake tanning options available now.

The benefits of fake tan

For those that want the look of a tan, without all the harmful effects, then fake tan is your friend.

The major benefit of choosing to use fake tan is that it's a lot safer than sunbathing or using a sunbed. You're not putting your skin at risk of premature ageing and, most of all, you're not increasing your risk of getting skin cancer.

Other benefits include the fact that you have full control over your fake tan application and can decide where on your body you'd like to use it and how much to use. Although sometimes it can take a few trials and errors to get it perfectly right – we've all heard horror stories of people turning out a nasty orange shade – you're ultimately able to get the tanning colour that you desire.

Tanning products have improved a lot over the years, thanks in part to the increased awareness of the dangers of sunbathing to get a tan, and most of the days of the ghastly orange disasters are over. In addition, if you don't fancy going through the motions of applying the fake tan yourself, there are now many tanning services on offer in beauty salons, where you pay someone else to apply it, or spray it on you.

Using fake tan

There are a lot of different brands of fake tan on the market and a variety of different ways in which they can be applied. Many come in bottles or sprays, ready to be applied in the privacy of your home.

The active ingredient in fake tan is something called dihydroxyacetone (DHA). When the product is put onto your skin, it reacts with the outer layer of the skin to produce the brown, tanned colour. It doesn't go beyond the outer layer of the skin, and isn't absorbed by the body.

Fake tan has to be reapplied regularly to maintain the look, because the outer skin cells are dead and naturally shed as the skin renews itself.

There are a lot of different tanning products available, but when you first buy a product it's advisable to test it on a small area of your skin before launching into using it properly. If you have an allergic reaction to it, then at least you'll know not to use the product. Likewise, if you're going to a tanning salon to be sprayed or painted with fake tan, then they should do a test on a patch of skin first.

'I used to use sunbeds when I was younger to get a tan and never thought skin cancer could happen to me. But at the age of 25 I got malignant melanoma.'

Emma.

Just remember that fake tan doesn't offer any sun protection abilities, so you'll still need to protect your skin from the sun with sunscreen if you're going to be outside.

Tanning moisturisers

In addition to fake tanning products, in recent years a number of tanning moisturisers have been developed too.

These products are designed to be used on a daily basis, perhaps for a few months over the summer or whenever you want to add colour to your skin, and help to gradually give your skin a tanned look over time. If you're not the biggest fan of traditional fake tan, and don't want the sudden effect that using fake tan can give, then slow-release tanning moisturisers may well appeal and can provide a healthy glow.

When you first start using them, you may not notice any change at all. But after you've used it for a while, you should start noticing subtle differences.

In addition to the subtle, slow, build-up effect that tanning moisturisers have, the other main benefit is that they're built into a moisturising product, which is of course good for your skin. As with fake tan, you still need to apply sunscreen too to get proper sun protection.

Checklist

- Don't be tempted to use a sunbed, especially if you're in a high risk group.
- Remember that a tan is a sign that the skin is damaged, not healthy.
- If you really want a tanned look, opt for fake tan.
- If you don't get on well with applying fake tan, consider visiting a salon.
- For a gradual tanned look, investigate the range of tanning moisturisers on the market.

Summing Up

- In addition to sunbathing being a major risk factor for skin cancer, using a sunbed can be very harmful too. Plus, it increases the risk of premature ageing.

- In fact, some sunbeds can emit UV rays that are 10-15 times stronger than those emitted from the midday sun.

- Every time you lie on a sunbed, the harmful effects of UV on your skin builds up and it is saved up over time.

- Anyone using a sunbed at least once a month or more increases their risk of skin cancer by 50%. Users of sunbeds who are aged under 35 increase their risk by 75%.

- Sunbed use in Scotland has been banned for the under 18s. Campaigning groups hope this will eventually be extended to the whole of the UK, especially as under 18s seem attracted to sunbeds.

- Neither using a sunbed nor lying out in the sun sunbathing are safe methods of tanning. In fact, a tan is really a sign that your skin has been damaged, not that it is healthy.

- If you really crave a tan, then the only safe method is to use fake tan.

- There are lots of fake tanning products available now that you can use yourself, or have applied by an expert.

- If you're not fond of traditional fake tan products, then a newer alternative is a tanning moisturiser. The effect is more subtle and builds up gradually over time.

Glossary

The ABCD Rule
A standard used by doctors that you can use to assess your moles for signs of changes. A stands for asymmetry, B for border, C for colour and D for diameter.

Basal cell carcinoma
The most common form of non-melanoma skin cancer in the UK. It starts in the deep basal cell layer of the epidermis, or the outer layer of the skin.

Biological therapy
A form of treatment that involves having an injection of interferon several times a week. The drug helps the body's immune system to fight the cancer.

Biopsy
A procedure which involves having a sample (in this case, of skin) removed so that it can be examined in depth under a microscope.

Broad-spectrum sunscreen
A term used to describe a sunscreen that offers protection against both UVB and UVA rays. The amount of UVB protection is measured by the SPF and the amount of UVA protection is determined by the UVA star system.

Carcinoma
Another word for cancer.

Chemotherapy
A form of cancer treatment that involves intravenous injections of drugs. With skin cancer, topical chemotherapy uses special creams applied to the affected area of the skin.

Cryotherapy or cryosurgery
A treatment for cancer that uses cold liquid nitrogen to destroy the cancer cells and tissues by freezing.

Curettage and cautery
A procedure where the cancer is scraped away (curettage) and then the skin is sealed up (cautery).

Dermatoscopy
A pain-free test that is sometimes used to analyse and magnify an area of suspect skin, prior to doing a biopsy. It involves the use of an instrument called a dermatoscope.

Dermis
The inner layer of the skin, where the sweat glands are located.

Epidermis
The elastic layer of skin on the outside, where melanin is produced.

Fake tan
A cosmetic beauty product that can be used to produce the colour and look of a tan, without the skin damage caused by sunbathing or using a sunbed.

Inorganic sunscreen

A type of mineral sunscreen that is designed to work like a mirror, reflecting the light away from the surface of the skin before it can get in.

Isolated limb perfusion

A technique that uses chemotherapy drugs to treat skin cancer that is isolated on a limb, such as an arm or leg. As the drug is only applied to that one limb, the side effects are not so bad.

Malignant melanoma

The most serious form of skin cancer. It's rare in children but has, worryingly, become the most common cancer for those aged 15 to 34 years old.

Melanin

Melanin is a pigment that gives the skin its colour. When the skin is exposed to sunlight, more melanin is produced as the skin tries to protect itself from UV radiation. This is what is known as getting a suntan.

Moles

Small dark marks that appear on the skin. They're usually circular or oval, and black or brown, but can be smooth, rough, raised, flat or hairy. Some people are born with moles, but they can also develop at any time

NICE

Acronym for the National Institute for Health and Clinical Excellence, an independent organisation providing guidelines about the prevention and treatment of ill health, and the promotion of good health.

Non-melanoma skin cancer

The most common type of skin cancer, accounting for about 100,000 cases in the UK each year. The main types of non-melanoma skin cancer are basal cell carcinoma and squamous cell carcinoma.

Organic sunscreen

A type of chemical sunscreen that works by absorbing the UV light on the surface of your skin, thus stopping the light from getting in.

Photodynamic therapy

A form of cancer treatment whereby a special light sensitising cream, injection or drug is used to make the skin sensitive to light. A laser light is then shone onto the affected area for a set period of time, killing off any cells that have been absorbed by the drug.

Radiotherapy

A form of treatment that uses high energy rays to destroy the cancer cells.

Skin flap

A complicated surgical procedure whereby a piece of tissue with its own blood supply (the skin and tissue beneath it) is removed from the donor site, close to the cancer wound, and reattached to the area of skin being repaired. It's usually used on scars that would be very noticeable after cancer surgery and it can provide a better result than a skin graft.

Skin graft

A surgical procedure where a piece of skin is taken from a donor site elsewhere on your body (usually in a place that isn't seen much, such as an inner thigh) and used to patch up the area where cancer has been removed.

Staging

A system used to help doctors and patients understand the size and stage of a tumour, and how far it's spread.

Squamous cell carcinoma

The second most common form of skin cancer in the UK. It starts in the outermost cells of the skin, when cells grow out of control and form a tumour. It grows at a faster rate than basal cell carcinoma.

Subcutaneous layer

A layer of the skin that is located under the dermis. It's made up of connective tissue and fat.

Sunbed

A device designed to produce UV radiation, mimicking the sun, under which people lie to gain a cosmetic tan.

Sunburn

Sunburn is a sign that the skin has been damaged. It's initially painful, inflamed and red, then the damaged skin peels away. But although the damaged layer is gone, the skin damage remains and can build up problems for the future.

Sunscreen

A specially designed skincare product that helps protect the skin from the harmful UVA and UVB rays emitted from the sun.

Sun protection factor (SPF)

A system used on sunscreens to help people know how much protection the individual product offers against the sun's UVB rays (the amount of UVA protection is measured by the UVA star system).

Tanning moisturiser

A cosmetic beauty product designed to produce the look of a tan over time. It has a more gradual effect than fake tan and is a safer method of adding colour to your skin than sunbathing or using a sunbed.

UV

Ultraviolet light or ultraviolet rays, which are emitted by the sun.

UVA

A long wavelength of UV radiation that is emitted by the sun. It can penetrate deep into the dermis, affecting the elastin of the skin, causing premature ageing and skin cancer.

UVA star system

A system used on sunscreen products to indicate how much protection the product gives against UVA. When used alongside SPF, a sunscreen is described as a broad-spectrum sunscreen.

UVB

A shorter wavelength of UV radiation emitted by the sun. It penetrates the epidermis, the upper layer of the skin, and can cause sunburn and skin cancer.

UVC

A type of UV radiation that can't get through the ozone layer, so it is not linked to skin damage or skin cancer.

UV index

A special index created by the World Health Organisation to measure the sun's rays. It is incorporated into many weather reports to show how strong the UV rays are. The higher the number, the greater the risk and the less time it takes for the sun to cause skin damage.

Vitamin D

A vitamin that is involved in helping build and maintain strong bones. The sun helps build up our vitamin D levels, but only a small amount of sun exposure is required.

Help List

American Academy of Dermatology
Address: P.O. Box 4014 Schaumburg, IL 60168-4014
Tel: (847) 240-1280
Contact form: https://www.aad.org/Forms/ContactUs/Default.aspx
Website: https://www.aad.org/
Info: Leading dermatological organisation, with a website full of useful resources.

British Association of Counselling and Psychotherapy
Address: British Association for Counselling and Psychotherapy, BACP House, 15 St John's Business Park, Lutterworth, Leicestershire, LE17 4HB, United Kingdom
Tel: 01455 883300
Email: bacp@bacp.co.uk
Website: http://www.bacp.co.uk/
Info: Provides a directory of qualified counsellors, which is updated each year, and they can help put you in touch with a counsellor in your area.

British Association of Dermatologists
Address: British Association of Dermatologists, Willan House, 4 Fitzroy Square, London, W1T 5HQ
Tel: +44 (0)207 383 0266
Email: admin@bad.org.uk
Website: http://www.bad.org.uk/
Info: The British Association of Dermatologists (BAD) is a charity whose charitable objects are the practice, teaching, training and research of Dermatology. It works with the Department of Health, patient bodies and commissioners across the UK, advising on best practice and the provision of Dermatology services across all service settings.

British Skin Foundation
Address: British Skin Foundation, 4 Fitzroy Square, London, W1T 5HQ
Tel: 0207 391 6341
Contact form: http://www.britishskinfoundation.org.uk/ContactUs.aspx
Website: http://www.britishskinfoundation.org.uk/
Info: Registered UK charity dedicated to skin research.

Cancer Active

Address: CANCERactive, Appletree Cottage, Hay Lane, Fulmer, Bucks, SL3 6HJ
Tel: 0300 365 3015
Email: admin@canceractive.com; wendy@canceractive.com
Website: http://www.canceractive.com/
Info: Cancer Active are a small UK charity devoted to empowering cancer sufferers to increase their personal odds of beating the disease. Their website also has a shop.

Cancer Research UK

Address: Cancer Research UK, Angel Building, 407 St John Street, London, EC1V 4AD
Tel: 020 7242 0200
Contact form: https://www.cancerresearchuk.org/about-us/contact-us/submit-a-question
Website: http://www.cancerresearchuk.org/
Info: Cancer Research UK are one of the leading UK fundraisers for cancer. Their website offers many useful resources, as well as information on how to get involved with fundraising.

Look Good, Feel Better

Address: Look Good Feel Better, West Hill House, 32 West Hill, Epsom, Surrey, KT19 8JD
Tel: 01372 747 500
Email: info@lgfb.co.uk
Website: http://www.lookgoodfeelbetter.co.uk/
Info: Free support service for women having treatment for cancer. They offer a unique programme of beauty workshops, with practical tips and advice for dealing with the visible side effects of treatment.

MacMillan

Address: Macmillan Cancer Support, 89 Albert Embankment, London, SE1 7UQ
Tel: 0808 808 00 00
Contact form: http://www.macmillan.org.uk/aboutus/contactus/askmacmillanform.aspx
Website: https://www.macmillan.org.uk/
Info: MacMillan are a leading cancer support charity in the UK, and their website offers access to useful information on various forms of cancer as well as fundraising.

Marie Curie Cancer Care

Address: Marie Curie, 89 Albert Embankment, London, SE1 7TP
Tel: 0800 090 2309
Online chat service: https://www.mariecurie.org.uk/help/marie-curie-support-line/using-online-chat
Website: https://www.mariecurie.org.uk/
Info: Organisation that runs hospices in the UK and provides nursing and care for patients in their own homes.

Met Office

Website: http://www.metoffice.gov.uk/
Info: Weather forecasting site where you can find the UV index predictions for your location.

National Council on Skin Cancer Prevention

Address: National Council on Skin Cancer Prevention c/o John Antonishak, Executive Director 1875 I Street, N.W., Suite 500 Washington, D.C. 20006
Tel: (301) 801 4422
Contact form: http://www.skincancerprevention.org/contact
Website: http://www.skincancerprevention.org/resources
Info: Website has a large number of links and resources which could come in useful.

Skin Cancer Foundation

Address: 149 Madison Avenue Suite 901 New York, NY 10016
Tel: (212) 725-5176
Contact form: http://www.skincancer.org/contact-us
Website: http://www.skincancer.org/
Info: Website has links to support resources here: http://www.skincancer.org/skin-cancer-information/support

The European Prospective Investigation into Cancer and Nutrition

Email: epic@iarc.fr
Website: http://epic.iarc.fr/
Info: EPIC was designed to investigate the relationships between diet, nutritional status, lifestyle and environmental factors and the incidence of cancer and other chronic diseases. EPIC is a large study of diet and health having recruited over half a million (520,000) people in 10 European countries: Denmark, France, Germany, Greece, Italy, The Netherlands, Norway, Spain, Sweden and the United Kingdom.

World Cancer Research Fund

Address: 22 Bedford Square, Fitzrovia, London WC1B 3HH

Tel: 0207 343 4200

Email: wcrf@wcrf.org

Website: https://www.wcrf-uk.org/

Info: The WCRF are similar to Cancer Research UK and others. They help sufferers and family through hard times, and raise money towards a cure.

Youth Cancer Trust

Address: Tracy Ann House, 5 Studland Road, Alum Chine, Bournemouth, BH4 8HZ

Tel: 01202 763 591

Email: admin@yct.org.uk

Website: http://www.youthcancertrust.org/

Info: Charity providing activity-based holidays for cancer sufferers aged 14 to 30.

Book List

ABC of Skin Cancer
By Sajjad Rajpar, John Wiley & Sons, Chichester, UK, 2008.

Beating Melanoma: A Five-Step Survival Guide
By Steven Q. Wang, Johns Hopkins UP, Baltimore MD USA, 2011.

The Cancer Survivor's Handbook
By Dr Terry Priestman, Sheldon Press, London, 2009.

Coping with Chemotherapy
By Dr Terry Priestman, Sheldon Press, London, 2005.

Coping with Radiotherapy
By Dr Terry Priestman, Sheldon Press, London, 2007.

Melanoma- Not Just Skin Cancer
By Catherine M Poole, Createspace, USA, 2015.

Understanding Chemotherapy
By Macmillan, London, 2009. (Available for free from publications.macmillan.org.uk)

Understanding Radiotherapy
By Macmillan, London, 2009. (Available for free from publications.macmillan.org.uk)

When Someone with Cancer is Dying
By Macmillan, London, 2007. (Available for free from publications.macmillan.org.uk)

When Someone You Love Has Cancer: A Guide to Help Kids Cope
By Alaric Lewis and R W Alley, One Caring Place, USA, 2005.